THE
NALINI METHOD

THE NALINI METHOD

TRANSFORM YOUR MIND AND BODY

7 WORKOUTS

FOR

7 MOODS

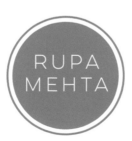

RUPA MEHTA

SEAL PRESS

Seal Press
A Member of the Perseus Books Group
1700 Fourth Street
Berkeley, California
sealpress.com

Library of Congress Cataloging-in-Publication Data on file.
ISBN 978-1-58005-599-4

10 9 8 7 6 5 4 3 2 1

Cover design by Erin Seaward-Hiatt
Interior design by Megan Jones Design
Photos by Will Haraldson, willharaldsonphoto.com, unless otherwise noted.

Printed in the United States of America
Distributed by Publishers Group West

This book is dedicated to you.

Thank you for choosing to spend your valuable time, effort, and energy on this book and its mission. I can offer the guidelines, workouts, and success stories, but that's only part of the journey—you bring the other piece to the table. It takes two, so thank you for being my other half.

CONTENTS

— INTRODUCTION —

My mother has always had a fondness for *daal*, an Indian lentil soup. Some of my most inspiring memories involve her grinding spices and cooking traditional Indian food for me in our homey kitchen. Our kitchen was filled with knick-knacks, my favorite being a plaque labeled "Mother's Rules." My mother, now seventy-five, is overweight, rendering her "unhealthy" by medical standards. But the sparkle in her eye, her self-awareness and resilience, her acceptance of life and who she is, and her calm and loving accumulated wisdom beg the question: What truly makes a person healthy? Is it your exercise routine? Is it what you eat? Is it your attitude? Is it your friends and family?

For me, the answer lies in one of the most unusual places, my mother's Sanskrit name, Nalini—the Hindi word for lotus. Hinduism and Buddhism see the lotus flower as a symbol for awakening to the spiritual reality of life. The lotus flower starts small, growing from the bottom of a body of water, like a pond, pushing through mud and muck. Only when it reaches the surface does the lotus bud begin to blossom into a beautiful flower.

So when it came time, twelve years ago, to name my business, calling it the Nalini Method was a no-brainer. Not only is my workout named after one of the healthiest people I know, my mom, but it also honors the journey of the lotus flower. This tough yet beautiful bloom reflects my favorite motto for life: *we're built to last*. Although the hard little bud of the lotus is bound by mud and dirt, as we are surrounded by life's challenges and messes, it still grows, thriving despite adversity, because it is built to last. It survives and so do we. Even if we experience physical struggles, unsupportive families or friendships, and unimaginable hardships, like the lotus we are innately built to survive and be our own teachers and healers.

It's difficult to objectively pinpoint what exactly makes you healthy. Some define it by body mass index, some by life expectancy, and some by happiness. I believe when you fully embrace the idea that you are your own best teacher and are in fact built to last, you reflect the type of health, vibrancy, and potential that go beyond physical limits. This kind of health is timeless, just like my mom's spirit.

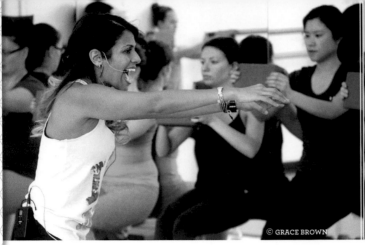
© GRACE BROWN

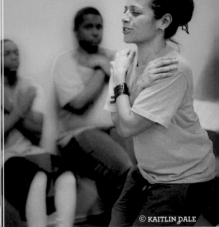
© KAITLIN DALE

It is this message that inspires my three-pronged approach to my adult classes and school program in New York City, where I guide my students to support and heal their own *minds*, *bodies*, and *hearts*.

The "mind/body connection" is a phrase frequently tossed around in the media, in schools, and in our own homes. Yet in the one place where the mind/body connection seems to be a natural fit—the world of fitness—the importance of the *body* workout still far outweighs the *mind* workout.

Why work out just one when you can so easily strengthen both at the same time? There are dozens of classes that fill us with endorphins for that much-craved high: spin classes that get us amped, dance classes that get us into the groove, meditative classes that soothe—but where are the workouts that equally address and challenge the mind as well as the body?

The answer lies in this book. As a fitness instructor for over fifteen years, I know that good physical fitness can never exist without good emotional fitness. If you're trying to be healthier physically, it's not just about the six-pack, perky butt, and the celeb-of-the-month arms. It's about admitting and owning up to your moods, about feeling confident, optimistic, resilient, and satisfied with your emotional life, too.

The Nalini Method will show you how to identify and allow you to manage not only your physical weight but your emotional weight as well. I like to call it a unique combination of mental and physical push-ups.

After all, understanding how to overcome a destructive and self-sabotaging mood by transforming your feelings is one of the greatest gifts you can give yourself. The better your mood is, the better your body feels; the better your body feels, the better your mood is. It's a cyclical and symbiotic process. If you can work out both your mind and your body consistently, you won't need to resort to extremes, like overly restrictive diets or dangerous workout routines, to make yourself feel better.

This is the premise of the Nalini Method: if you can develop a reliable and internally balanced emotional and physical core foundation, you can *always* make yourself feel better physically. You won't have to starve yourself and guzzle raw juices that cost more than a pair of shoes, or jump on fad diets, or dedicate your life to yoga or meditation, intensive bodybuilding, or boot camp classes every day. Instead, you'll be able to draw upon this steady, firm foundation to give you the strength you're craving, no matter what the situation.

How the Nalini Method Came to Be

I started the Nalini Method because I saw an enormous void in the fitness world. I wanted to develop a simple, highly accessible, preventive wellness system with great personalized potential and effectiveness, a workout that is as active emotionally as it is physically. It's a system with long-lasting effects: results that can be felt outside of your workout time and spill into your relationships and life. It tackles emotional and physical weight head-on and places an even degree of importance on both.

PHYSICAL AND EMOTIONAL WEIGHT

It's important to reaffirm that you can be physically fit yet still emotionally overweight, just as you can be emotionally fit and physically overweight. Our society's idea and definition of weight are unbalanced. With an obsessive focus on only physical weight and a disregard for our emotional well-being, even the most popular fitness books, products, and services can do a disservice to their audience. My goal is to support you on your journey to not only becoming physically fit but also feeling emotionally fit. You will gain confidence and lose *true* weight (both physical and emotional), when you do the Nalini Method regularly.

To truly transform and connect to our lives, we must rethink weight. The kind of weight loss that I know would benefit my clients, the kids I teach, and anyone looking to live their life to the best of their abilities requires something beyond physical exercise and diet. It requires an emotional diet as well.

After all, while there is no objectively perfect body, mind, or person, there is a perfect *you.* Maybe you like to be full-figured or maybe you like to be thin—none of it matters if your spirit is weighed down. A healthy person isn't weighed down by emotions. Instead, their true spirit shines so clearly and vibrantly that the world can't help but experience it.

So, rather than chase after the subjective notions of body and mind prescribed to us, let's reevaluate our ideals through a different lens of health. By rethinking weight, we can physically and emotionally trim down to discover the light, beautiful, and individual bodies and spirits that naturally live within us.

This book is not about feeling happy, giddy, and on top of the world twenty-four hours a day, seven days a week—that's impossible! What I hope to teach you is how to recognize and appreciate a true mind/body connection, with workouts that specifically address your mood in the moment. They will allow you to mitigate the overwhelming effects of a negative mood, or capitalize on the benefits of a positive one. This will not only improve your resilience, like that of the lotus and my mother, but give you the tools to lose both emotional and physical weight and live a lighter, healthier life.

It doesn't matter who my students are—fit, strong, flexible, and lean adults or adolescents who think a crunch is a sugary breakfast cereal—I can instantly tell who in my classes is fully present. I can also tell who is letting their feelings get in the way of an optimal workout. Heavy emotional weight can pull you down and make you more likely to get sick, fail at relationships, and lose trust, patience, and tolerance. It can create a diminished sense of self, self-acceptance, self-esteem, self-control, and presence. Your state of mind emanates from your physical body: from where you choose to focus your eyes, to being fidgety and anxious, to where and how you give up in an exercise, to how you wear your outfit, to how you respond to your instructor. Inevitably, your body will reflect your mind. When you can see that excess, unresolved emotional weight can be just as detrimental as excess physical weight, you can choose to find a way to shed it and drive your mind and body to feel free and light. You can shine to your fullest potential and enjoy a more effective workout.

Like everyone, I have those difficult, can't-get-out-of-that-mood kinds of days. Normally, I bounce out of bed at 6 a.m., eager to get my busy day going. I drink a fresh vegetable juice, eat a banana, have a cup of yogurt, and go teach my classes with a kick in my step. Other days, forget it. I feel like I'm walking through mud and every minute feels like ten. A fresh green smoothie? No way: hand over the bacon and cold leftovers from the night before. I'm dragging. I do *want* to feel better, but just can't. I go through the motions knowing full well that an optimum mindset and workout just aren't going to happen.

Yet even on the crummiest of crummy days, I know that I will wake up the next day and start over again. Even if I want to be locked in my small apartment with a flashing neon DO NOT DISTURB sign over my door (which is turned off only for food deliveries from my favorite restaurant's takeout guy), that mood will pass because

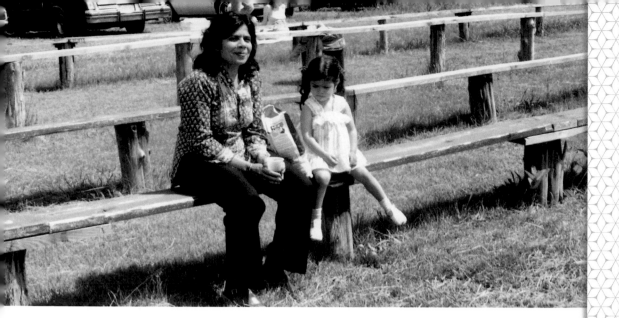

I am built to last, and because I know how to manage my emotional weight as well as my physical weight.

One of my favorite quotes is from Galileo: "You cannot teach a man anything; you can only help him find it within himself." The aim of this book is not only to encourage but also to enable this critical access to your best inner teacher. Your confidence will build quickly as you start to manage your moods better and experience wonderful physical changes in your body. And before you know it, you will relish in knowing that you are in fact your best teacher, your best healer, and you are built to last.

How the Nalini Method Works

This book is divided into three parts, allowing you to uncover and verbalize the specific mood you are in so you can then use your emotions as a tool to better understand, strengthen, and nourish your body.

In Part I, Chapter 1, I cover the vital distinction between emotional and physical weight. This understanding is the powerful lens that reveals what being healthy, confident, and happy truly means. You'll learn about the ultimate mind/body connection and the dynamic and essential foundation upon which the Nalini Method is built. You'll see how to own up to your moods, and you'll quickly come to understand why this mood-based system is so effective. In Chapter 2, you'll be given all the fundamentals needed to best approach and reap the benefits of all the different workouts.

In Part II, the workout party begins! Depending on your mood, you can choose from any of the seven mood workouts: *Anger, Energy, Stress, Chill, Happiness, Doubt,* and *Anxiety.*

What makes this book unique is that each of the seven routines will provide you with an optimal workout no matter how you're feeling—as if you have your own trainer in the privacy of your home. Each workout addresses not only the emotional component of your mood but the physical actions that best suit it. For example, when you're chill you may feel relaxed and a bit lazy, so you need gentler starting movements. But with anger, you know you need to move right away. So, if you're feeling good, you'll feel even better and if you're feeling bad, these workouts will click you out of a downhill state of mind and jump-start your life engine.

Have you ever been in a yoga class when you're angry or anxious and have not been able to focus? You might have even come out of class frustrated that you wasted an hour or didn't get the kind of workout you wanted. Sometimes your true intention is not to zen out in yoga but to have the space to experience your mood without feeling pressured to be positive.

You don't have to worry about that kind of situation again, because these workouts are tailored to *your* needs. Because you're choosing the workout that best suits your mood in the moment, you will be able to give it your full attention and get the results you're craving. These workouts will provide:

- a strong mind/body connection
- a sculpted and stronger physique
- longer and leaner muscles
- enhanced flexibility and balance
- improved body awareness, posture, and alignment
- increased bone density
- increased endurance and energy

In Part III, you'll learn how to super-charge your Nalini Method workouts to make them even more effective, with healthy ideas and juice recipes rooted in the ancient principles of Ayurvedic medicine.

The Nalini Method is a challenging, practical, fun, and intuitive path to tap into the tools already within you to transform your mind and your body. Once you decide to *own* your mood, you can make it work *for* you. I want you to consider this book your toolbox as well as your support system on your journey to becoming your own best teacher and healer.

PART I
THE NALINI METHOD

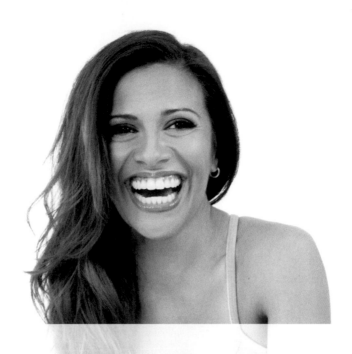

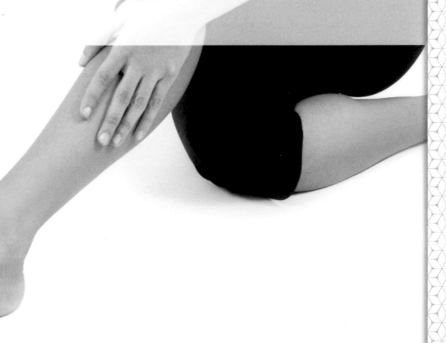

---------- CHAPTER 1 ----------

THE NALINI METHOD
MIND/BODY CONNECTION

You can be fit *and* unhealthy. You can be thin *and* large. You can be heavy *and* light. You can be physically in shape *and* emotionally out of shape. You can be mentally strong *and* physically weak.

You've seen it and likely experienced it: slim, toned, and fit men and women, young and old, from all different backgrounds, working in a wide range of careers, looking at their flat bellies, firm thighs, and killer bodies with no sparkle in their eyes. They may have the toned legs you've dreamed about but lack a kick in their step. Whatever is pressing on them emotionally seems to pack an additional hundred pounds onto their shoulders. Even if they have little body fat anywhere to be seen, the weight of their emotions makes them *feel* fat.

And you've probably also seen unfit or overweight men and women, young and old, from all different backgrounds, looking at their big booties and curvier bodies with glowing confidence in their eyes. They may not fit into the top model mold, but they don't care—they have an undeniable and contagious swagger. Although their attitude is like a balloon lifting them up from feeling weighed down, their extra fifty pounds of body fat still makes them physiologically overweight.

I am so heavy. I feel fat. I am fat. I weigh so much. I need to lose weight.

In the world of fitness, I hear these loaded words so often and from people of all shapes and sizes that I was inspired to look up the dictionary definition of the word "weight."

What I found intrigued me. According to the *New Oxford American Dictionary*, weight is "the heaviness of a person or thing." Pounds and physical mass are not even mentioned. This, I realized, is society's interpretation of weight. That's when it clicked: no matter how much a person works out, if they are emotionally overweight, they will feel and demonstrate the exact same symptoms of being and feeling physically heavy.

Both our bodies and our minds have weight to them. What makes our bodies healthy is nutritious food and exercise. What make our minds healthy is nutritious words and actions.

Despite being physically in shape, I've been emotionally out of shape at various points in my life, and I'm sure you have, too. These are the times when you feel the weight of the world. You have trouble taking charge of your life. You may feel so stressed-out that you can only see problems, and because solutions aren't on the horizon, these problems seem to grow larger and larger. There might be movement in your body but no movement in your thoughts.

If I asked you, "When you think of the word 'fat,' what comes to mind?" many of you would answer, "Lazy, slow, large, lacking in energy and motion, *stuck*." When you are emotionally out of shape and overweight you feel the same effects of being physically overweight. You feel *stuck*. Stuck in a mood that is increasing in size, making you *feel* fat. Making you *act* fat.

What makes us feel fat, stuck, and lacking in confidence is not just our bodies; it's the situations and relationships in our lives. It's the weight of the situations and relationships we may not know how to navigate or change. It's easier to choose the quick fixes, like drinking, smoking, emotional eating, or avoidance, to help us manage these situations. Yet these untenable solutions just continue to increase our physical and emotional weight. If we could all step on a scale that measures emotional weight, I think many of us would be shocked. We have no idea how much our unaddressed emotions can add to any discouraging heaviness and weight in our lives.

We *can* lose this emotional weight—and that's where this book can transform your life. Your mind requires different exercises than your body, and your body will perform exercises better with a stronger mind. The Nalini Method workouts work the mind and body in unison, enabling you to efficiently lose both emotional and physical weight. By making optimal use of your time and giving way to quicker and better results, you will create a balanced, lighter, and healthier life.

The ultimate mind/body connection is about getting to that deeply satisfying place where your emotional weight and physical weight are in perfect balance. When you feel good about your mind and body, you feel good about your life. You feel *whole*. You're more confident and able to follow your heart, leading you to a better life, full of passion and full of possibilities.

If, however, your mind is in a great place but your body isn't, or vice versa, your confidence level plummets and your ability to see hopeful possibilities diminishes. When that happens, you will find that a Nalini Method mood workout will click you out of that mindset. These mood-driven workouts force you to accept who you are and the validity of all your feelings, to acknowledge your emotional weight, and to own it. When you own your emotional weight, you can stop and reverse that downhill avalanche or enhance a great zone and empower your complete self.

I wish that the term "weight" would inextricably intertwine both "emotional weight" and "physical weight." You can't lose physical weight efficiently if you don't exercise, and you can't exercise efficiently if you don't lose the heaviness of your unaddressed emotional weight. Emotional weight is the thundercloud that can keep you from getting into the zone.

As human beings, we all have tools to help us navigate our lives. We have our emotional mind, our physical body, and our spiritual heart that keep us going. When these tools are disconnected, we can't function at our optimum strength and potential. Until we recognize and articulate what our emotional weight is, and how leaving it unaddressed makes our mind/body connection out of whack, we will never achieve our ideal physical weight and become truly in shape.

Measuring Emotional Weight

There is no scale to measure emotional weight, so we need to develop a method of making it as tangible as physical weight. If we can start to see it, we can start to manage it. The symptoms of being emotionally overweight are anger, anxiety, depression, doubt, inability to visualize and plan for future goals, lack of effective communication skills, lack of physical movement, lack of self-control, and stress. The Mind/Body Equivalents chart below provides a way to make emotional weight a palpable reality so we can begin to evaluate and manage it as we do physical weight.

MIND/EMOTIONAL	BODY/PHYSICAL
Words: Digested into your soul	**Foods**: Digested into your body
Playlists: What gets added to your thoughts	**Pounds**: What gets added to your body
Actions: Keep your mind fit	**Exercise**: Keeps your body fit
Aura: How you are perceived by the world	**Appearance**: How you look to the world
Charting: Measures your emotional weight	**Scale**: Measures your physical weight

WORDS

How we understand, articulate, and share ourselves with the world occurs through words. If you were asked to describe how you feel in ten words, the words you'd pick would reflect your emotional weight. And, of course, we all have different interpretations of words; the word "happy" may bear different weight for me than it does for you. The word "fearful" may feel different to me than to you. The *weight of words* is unique to each of us, depending on our individual life experiences.

Over the years, we've all accumulated the weight of words. Just as we should be aware of what we eat for our bodies, we should also be aware of the exact words we digest into our minds. One word has the power to weigh us down much more than a single scoop of ice cream, or to lift us up like fresh-squeezed orange juice. There are healthy and unhealthy words, just as there are healthy and unhealthy foods that make you gain or lose physical pounds.

Our minds and bodies go through daily fluctuations of weight, energy, and hormones. Some of these are controlled by you, what you eat, or what's going on in your life, and some are triggered by your natural hormonal fluctuations or are out of your control. How you piece together words that are in your control and out of your control (other people's words that you listen to) become the thoughts and sayings you live with and by. Who do you think shares the most words with you? Trick question . . . It's *you*! You hang out with yourself all day long, and it is the words, thoughts, and sayings you listen to that affect your mood the most.

PLAYLISTS

I like to think of our minds as powerful mp3 players/iPods. Our mind is a stereo system in surround sound, providing us with little but loud voices all day long. We have different "songs" that we listen to internally: songs that lift us up or bring us down, songs that make us angry or that trigger blissful memories. Our playlist is the compilation of songs we choose to listen to; it's the most important music we play in our lives. More simply, this playlist acts as our conscience, the compilation of words or thoughts in our head, which tell us who we will be in that moment, throughout the day, or for the rest of our lives. The playlist you choose can be the very voices in your head that keep your life in harmony or get you completely out of tune.

For example, I have a doubtful song in my mind called "Who the hell am I to try to change things?" I also have a hopeful song in my mind, which is one of my favorite quotes: "If you think you're too small to make a difference in the world, you haven't been in bed with a mosquito." It's my choice to pick the song that gets the most play.

The concept of an internal playlist and the value of a strong conscience came from my father, who has had quite an inspiring life. He was born in India, on a boxcar of a noisy freight train, the second-to-last of nine siblings. His unusual birthplace came about because my grandfather was desperately poor and worked on the tracks, so the entire family lived on a train transporting materials between the jungles and villages of India. When he was a child, my father had to worry about poisonous snakes crawling across him at night, having enough food to share with all his brothers and sisters, and trying to get clean clothes to wear. He did not grow up with access to dreams that could easily become a reality. He attended fourteen different schools, and had to start working at a very young age. Any money he made went to support his family.

Based on his experiences, it would have been easy for him to identify himself as a poor, uneducated boy or a lost cause. But from an early age, my dad identified himself as rich in experiences, educated in common sense, entitled to formal schooling, and adaptable. He somehow managed to put himself through school in India, get a green card, and come to America with only $8 in his pocket. That was forty years ago. To give you a sense of the culture shock he initially faced, the first time he went to a restroom in America, he went there to rest. He fell asleep on a chair because, after all, it was called a *rest*room.

Thanks to his healthy emotional weight and strong self-identity, he was able to adapt to his new experiences in a new country. He made the decision not to just learn but to master the English language. He made the decision to work hard and become one of the first Indian American lawyers practicing in Washington, D.C., at that time. He made the decision to settle down in one home, in one neighborhood, for over thirty years, so his children would never experience being uprooted multiple times as he was, living in the boxcars of India.

My dad's mental playlist is one of the best I've ever heard. His most played song is "No one can take away your happiness," and is the inspiration for Chapter 8. It helps him bounce back, whether from the people who mocked him for sleeping in the restroom or for his Indian accent, his song helps him keep his emotional weight balanced and harmonious.

You certainly can't change your past, but you can always change your mental playlist and, by doing so, your future. On any given day, before you even eat breakfast, you've probably started packing on emotional weight. Let's say you wake up in the morning and tell yourself, "I have to have a good day and be positive," or "I will only be happy when I lose weight," or "I'm so beautiful, nothing can bring me down." With these thoughts, you've already started constructing your playlist for the day. Part of the Nalini Method is to unveil this metaphorical iPod and drive your inner DJ to pump the jams and create playlists that work for you. Choose your playlists wisely, with variety to keep you in sync and balanced. You can always benefit from downloading a new playlist, literally and figuratively, one that reflects your current situation and aspirations.

Just as unhealthy physical pounds will make your body heavier, unhealthy mental playlists will make your mind heavier. Just as you cut down on junk food and sugar when you want to lose physical weight, you can cut down on the words and playlists

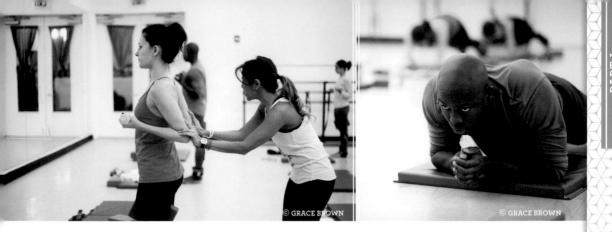

© GRACE BROWN   © GRACE BROWN

that don't work for you too. Replace them instead with words and thoughts that make you feel mentally nourished. In Part II, I introduce mood workout mantras that will be healthy songs to add to your playlist.

Bottom line: For many of us, it can often feel impossible to escape what's going on in our heads. When that happens, you need a process that brings movement to your stagnant thoughts, which can then translate to natural and transformative body movement. These mood mantras help you do just that, by allowing your mind to listen and move freely to fresh new "music."

ACTIONS

Words and playlists eventually lead to mental action—your mind's exercise. It takes actions of both mind and body to lose true weight. For many of us, going for a thirty-minute run outside is much easier than devoting thirty minutes to a mental or emotional workout. For example, making a phone call to own up to the words we said to a loved one in a fight is often much harder than going on that run. But it's the phone call workout that will ultimately help us lose that emotional weight.

With the Nalini Method, if you're angry and choose to complete the Anger workout, you might be telling yourself afterward, "I either need to let go or have an honest conversation about this." You might even be compelled to turn this mental movement into the very actions that affect your emotional weight.

If you begin to be aware of and visualize emotional weight in a practical way, it will affect your daily behavior and eventually transform your life. Just as making tiny changes in your diet and exercise helps chip away at physical weight, the same thing occurs with emotional weight. Eliminating just one negative word or destructive playlist from your soul diet could be all it takes to ignite emotional weight loss. When you understand your current emotional diet, the words and playlists you've accumulated over the years, you can successfully change and create emotional actions that lead you to a healthier life.

When you're having one of those impossible days at work, you will now be able to tell yourself, "Well, I hate push-ups, but I can do ten now in perfect form. I didn't think I could ever get strong arms, and now look at me. I did it. I didn't think I could ever observe and quantify my mood, and now I love to. I do a self-check every day. I did it. I can accomplish a seemingly unattainable goal. And I can make it through the next ten minutes or ten hours. This too shall pass. I can cope; I'm built to last."

We all want to be able to enter that confident place of feeling light and losing weight. But the path there takes much more than an incredible physical workout; it takes incredible emotional actions as well. It requires actions of strength and conviction to challenge the exclusive ideas of pounds, food, exercise, and perfection that intermingle so seamlessly in the health world. You have to embrace who you are first, emotionally *and* physically, to successfully go somewhere new. The act of owning up to your mood will transform your actions, weight, and aura much more than you can imagine.

AURA

The weight of your words, playlists, and actions manifests in your physical appearance through your demeanor, energy, and vibrancy. In other words, your aura is the physical part of your emotional weight. It's why I can tell who in my classes has emotional weight that is making them *appear* heavy. That's why my friends can tell if I feel heavy even if I've been working out hard. Your seemingly elusive aura is that visible!

I can have really bad moods and days when I want to lock myself in my bedroom and cry for hours. But even if I wake up like that, my clients will always be met with a genuine smile and a palpably pleasing aura because I know how to find the balance and resilience to keep my emotional weight in check. I have learned how to put my mood on hold or into perspective. When I own my feelings and mood, I am in charge of them. I've also learned that my sad mood can in fact still drive an effective, personalized workout. After all, there is nothing worse than feeling down in the dumps in your mind and letting your body go as a result because you can't muster up enough energy to work out—all while knowing you're giving off an aura that you wouldn't even want to hang out with! That's why it's so important to understand all the elements of emotional weight, including how you are perceived (by others as well as by yourself), so you can make a better plan for when you wake up on the wrong side of the bed!

CHARTING

Charting is the first step to achieving and maintaining ideal emotional weight. Let's face it: it is very hard, if not impossible, to fully quantify our emotional weight. You could, for example, have a "light" happiness (1 on the scale) if it's attached to celebration and triumph as well as a "heavy" (10 on the scale) happiness if it's attached to guilt or loss. You can even have a "light" anger if it's attached to humor or perseverance. Charting honestly is key and it takes a bit of practice. Better accuracy and charting lead to stronger self-awareness.

By charting we can start to quantify the factors that *create* our emotional weight, and we will be able to evaluate and eventually balance the words, songs, playlists, and resulting aura that affect it. Just as jumping on a scale can start the calculated, accountable path to physical weight loss, charting can ignite an empowering and responsible journey to emotional weight loss. Recording the weight of your mood over time will help you regulate your emotional weight and typical fluctuations.

When first incorporating this new measurement into your life, you may find it helpful to chart every day for a month. Simply match your emotional weight to a number on a scale between 1 (light) and 10 (heavy). Over time you will gain insight into your natural rhythm and how your feelings and mood fluctuate.

THE EMOTIONAL SCALE

In general, I am not a fan of stepping on a scale every day. Nor am I a fan of charting every day, because I know how much a person's weight can fluctuate. But different life events warrant different approaches. Sometimes, you will feel the need to use the emotional scale every day for a week or even a month, and other times you may not need it at all.

```
        1                        5                        10
     Light                   Neutral                    Heavy
```

When you're in a bad mood, you may feel as if it lasts for ages and will never go away. If you chart your moods, however, you'll get a clearer idea of what moods affect you the most, and how often. You'll see how things might average out more than you thought they did, and that your emotional weight is actually very stable and balanced. Or, you might see patterns that allow you to identify certain mood triggers—the grumpy receptionist at your office on Fridays, the traffic on the way to the grocery store, funny emails from your grandmother, and countless others—that you can work to either mitigate or multiply.

An easy way to chart reliably is by implementing a morning or evening check-in. Look at yourself in a mirror and ask, "What is my emotional weight?" Stating such a straightforward question is a wonderful way to own your feelings.

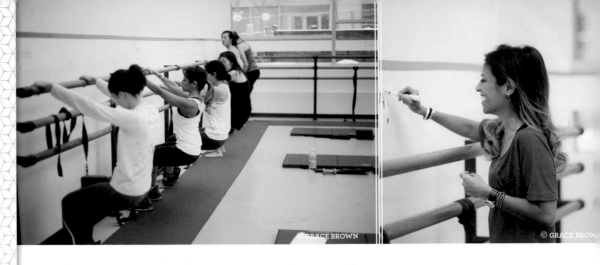

© GRACE BROWN

© GRACE BROWN

Managing Your Emotional Weight

Have you ever been sold the promise that if you work out and have a killer body, then you'll be happy and have a great life? I'm sure you have. I know this can work for some people, but for others, it just doesn't.

Similarly, have you ever had someone tell you what to feel? A person in your life may say something like, "That shouldn't bother you, just let it go," or "You should be happy." Doesn't that make you feel heavy? Of course it does! It doesn't feel natural to give up ownership of your weight or moods.

The more you own your moods, the more you'll see your own emotional weight clearly and succinctly. You're entitled to your own feelings and moods, even the dark ones! If you fully own your mood, whether you're furious or ecstatic, it will be totally genuine. You're being who you are instead of who you're told to be. And as your day goes by, you'll see and eventually accept how your unique emotional weight actually fluctuates due to various circumstances.

Your goal is not to eliminate your mood or how you feel. A healthy emotional weight is about *awareness* of your feelings. With this awareness comes the realization that your feelings can be addressed. That openness to new thoughts already lightens the load. It's why you state your mood at the beginning and end of each workout in Part II. You may start out stressed but turn out to be a bit less stressed after doing the Stress workout. And by chosing to do the workout you have *owned* this stress. You took what could have become a *stuck* mind filled with rigid thoughts and chose to *move* it instead. You have the power now, not the stress. Owning and working out your mood are what give you a healthy emotional weight.

These baby steps—acknowledging your mood and charting—give you the tools you need to fine-tune your mental playlist. In my classes, no one likes push-ups. (Well . . . maybe a handful of students do!) But we all know, the more you do them, the better you get at them. You build up your strength slowly, and before you know it your body can change and you can achieve something you never thought you could do. (Even if you still hate doing them!) Think of owning your mood as performing a mental push-up and you will get stronger with time and appreciate transformative benefits.

When you think of emotional weight in this hands-on way, you'll realize that very little mind work can go a very long way. By using the emotional scale, you can consciously introduce thoughts that encourage you to balance both your emotional and physical weight—ultimately shifting the scale in a lighter direction.

Losing fifty pounds is incredibly difficult and takes months, even years, of concerted effort. But it is possible, if you are committed. After you accomplish the big goal, it becomes about mindful maintenance. Sometimes it takes hard work to *not* have to work. Although the physical work may be over, you still have to deal with who you are, what your words and actions are, and how you *feel* to be able to upgrade to that confident lifestyle. Once you strive for healthy emotional weight and develop the Nalini Method mind/body connection, you'll see that you can successfully address your happiness and manage your weight in a whole new way.

CARLOS'S STORY

When I met Carlos, one of my middle-school students, he was fragile, uncoordinated, and desperately shy. He never looked his teacher in the eye or raised his hand in class. But when I told him about Chapter 3's mantra, "The solution is born before the problem," I saw a spark in his eye. This mantra is one of the hardest to understand, let alone fully accept. Carlos drew great comfort from knowing he was the first student for whom this mantra clicked. He was truly able to see the world as being filled with solutions instead of problems.

Before I knew it, this little boy was cranking out thirty push-ups, because his size was no longer an obstacle for him. He felt strong in his mind, and that mind could drive and create a strong body. At the end of our program, he got up in front of his class—head high and making eye contact with everyone—and said that the one word that defined him was "creative." Harnessing a unique word that could act as a compass for his day allowed him to move in new directions, opening up new possibilities. From heavy to light, his aura had completely changed, solely by recognizing the *weight of words* and changing the playlists and mantras in his head.

His teacher and classmates were astonished at his transformation. Carlos was living proof of the Chapter 3 mantra. His creativity led him to a world filled with inspiring solutions.

Mind/Body Connection: Emotional Weight/ Physical Weight Connection

If you took a survey asking people about the mind/body connection, I'll bet that many of them would give one of two responses. Some might say, "If I have positive thoughts and a great body, then I will figure out everything and my life will be better." Others might say, "If I'm stressed-out emotionally, then I'll be stressed out physically, too."

The Nalini Method mind/body connection is different. It goes like this: my actual weight is a reflection of both my emotional and physical weight. A healthy connection between my emotional and physical weight requires ownership of my moods, which will dictate the kind of life I choose to create for myself. When I own up to who I am—good, bad, and everything in between—I am forced to have movement in my mind that will dictate my connection to the world.

Many people assume that a mind/body connection can only be achieved on a yoga mat or during meditation, and that you must have a positive mindset in order to be emotionally healthy. But when your emotional weight is balanced, even if you're having the worst day ever, you'll be able to focus and/or realign yourself through a healthy lens on any goal.

Being fully present and at peace with yourself—without any pressure to feel a certain way or to present a certain face because you think it's expected of you—is a much easier goal to strive for than many of the other goals we set for ourselves. Through this system, you will have the space to give equal weight to the angry mood and the chill mood. But you won't be thinking of anger as always bad and chill as always good. It's like cholesterol: you have good and bad levels, and ideally they keep each other in check. You don't want to be depressed all day long but you don't want to be high on life every second either. We shouldn't feel as if we need to dedicate our lives to always feeling light, because *all* moods make the world go round, even anger. You just want to be striving for that balance where you are comfortable owning up to the things you say and do.

We can have a lot of different things going on in any given moment. The other day I was stressed and happy at the same time. That might sound paradoxical, but it wasn't, because I had fully accepted all of my feelings, good and bad. And by choosing and acknowledging your "leading" mood to even begin a workout, you are forced to become fully aware of your mind/body connection and own it.

When we're sensibly trying to lose weight or get in shape, we know it won't happen in one day. We give ourselves a long rope and small, consistent expectations. Just as you won't lose twenty pounds overnight, you won't be able to balance your emotional weight overnight. But you can start to reappraise yourself, emotionally and physically, once you own your moods and respect a new kind of mind/body balance.

After all, when you know how to do a push-up, your form is better. When you know how your mind works, you'll have the awareness to manage your thoughts and mood with more power and clarity. Those who come to my classes know I hold them accountable for working hard with their bodies and their minds. I trust them to do this and they reward my trust by accepting the challenge. My confidence in them is contagious and fuels their own confidence.

You can get that very same confidence using this book. When you finish the workouts in Part II, that Nalini Method mind/body connection will follow you off the mat and into all aspects of your life.

Living the Nalini Method: Mind/Body-Heart-World Connection

Appreciating the role and power of our own emotional weight can lead us to better manage the "weight" of the world.

The Nalini Method is rooted in the belief that the ultimate mind/body connection leads you to a *heart* connection and then a *world* connection. With a clear mind and strong body you'll have the space, energy, and desire to listen to your heart and live out your purpose, strengths, and passions. That is your *heart* connection. When you're doing the work your heart wants to do, ultimately it affects you and others in a wonderfully positive way. It's that web of positivity and connectivity that makes the world a better, more accountable place, as you live and delight in a *world* connection.

A greater mind/body connection puts you in the mood to delve deeper, go further, and have a happier and more fulfilling life that affects others.

This book is filled with the practical, fundamental, and crucial steps needed to live out your greatest potential. It will help you push past whatever has added to your emotional and physical weight—because, as you know, when you are stuck in mind or body, it's hard to have room for thoughts like "What's my purpose?" or "What will make me happy?" let alone "How can I contribute to the world?" Those questions are possible to answer, but it all starts with the first step: *you.*

I am a breast-cancer survivor, and when I went to Rupa's class it was my first attempt at exercising in a very long time. My thoughts were a jumble. I was so afraid and concerned yet happy to be alive.

Before class started, Rupa introduced herself and then asked me if I had any health concerns that might mean modifying some of the exercises. I wondered if I should say anything about my cancer but quickly realized it would be silly not to, as I could end up hurt. When I told Rupa I had survived breast cancer, all she said was, "Oh, congratulations," with a warm smile and in a very matter-of-fact way. There was no pity in her voice. She treated me like everyone else, not as a victim, and I felt lighter right away because she had acknowledged *me* without it being about my cancer. Her attitude was stunning. She had so brilliantly accentuated the positive with those two little words, and at that instant everything changed for me. I felt so lucky to be there.

Because there was so much spillage from me feeling so emotionally fragile into my feelings about my body, Rupa opened up my attitude to physical activity in a whole new way. She was never about pointing out what I couldn't do. She was only about what I could achieve and how much I was improving from one class to the next. I never had to deal with the emotional weight of thinking I had to be the healthiest or the skinniest person in the class. If we were told to do twenty reps, for example, and I could only do four, then rest, and then do two more, she'd never tell me I was "cheating." She praised me for trying my best and encouraged me to make a quick comeback when I stopped to rest.

It is not hyperbole for me to say that I owe my healing to Rupa. Her encouragement shut my inner critic right down! The stronger I got physically, the stronger I got emotionally. I now feel confident and healthy. She has such a light about her, and is such a source of energy, that she always makes me feel empowered. And, if *she* sees me this way, then I *am* strong and accomplished, and I can only get stronger. Her method is not about how far you have to go, but how much you've already accomplished.

You can actually accomplish all the healthy things your heart desires. But you have to start with you. Your mood could change your body, your body could change your mood, your mood affects your life's drive, and what you decide to do with your life can affect the world. It is truly all connected. Establishing a healthy emotional weight and a Nalini Method mind/body connection is the bridge leading you to marvelous connections with the world.

I encourage you to visualize yourself as someone who is built to last, like the lotus. Read and use this book as if we were working out together. Use the Nalini Method to maintain your ideal emotional and physical weight and improve your moods, and to strengthen your mind, body, and heart. You have the tools, so come and join me on the rewarding journey to shape our minds, bodies, and, as a result, our world.

My Personal Note to You

I'm thrilled and honored that you have chosen to pick up this book and share your time with me. I wish I could meet you in person, as I pride myself on being an individualized and personal teacher even when my classes are filled to capacity. For me, there is nothing like a real-time connection. Even though we are not meeting in person, I am writing from the heart. It's contagious: The more I own up, the more you'll own up. The more you own up, the better the results. Awareness is the first step to empowerment, after all.

So own your emotions. Own your words and actions. Own your movements. Own your body. Own your intentions. Owning all the physical moves you make during your workout will give you a true mind/body connection. Use these workouts as your sacred time for yourself—the one part of your day when you truly own your mood and are present emotionally and physically, and when you fully accept and embrace who you are and how you feel, with no distractions and no interruptions. Once you embody and own this mind/body connection, you start to unlock your greatest potential.

As I say in the beginning of each one of my classes: "You have chosen to be here, so *be* here, make our time special and effective!"

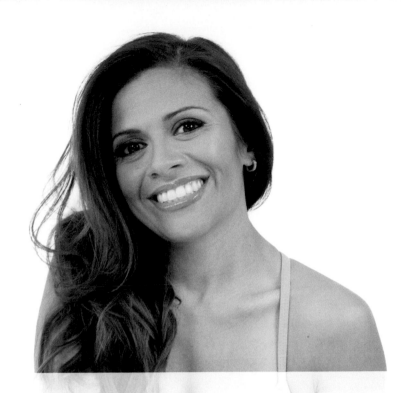

CHAPTER 2
THE FUNDAMENTALS

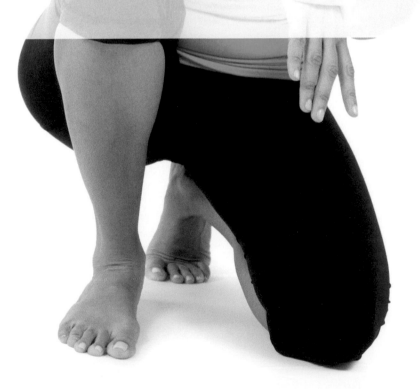

I see our initial interaction—before the actual exercising officially starts—as the *most* important part of the Nalini Method. It allows us to build a space of support and trust. As a result, you'll feel more comfortable with my method, and I'll feel more comfortable and trusted to guide you along the way.

My clients and I take this trust seriously. They expect me to look out for and take care of them during class. They've given me unspoken permission to hold them accountable and help them with form. They expect that I will not single them out unnecessarily but will make them feel special. They expect the attention and results of a personal trainer in a group class atmosphere. They expect the confidence, openness, and respect of a successful teacher. They expect their minds and bodies will feel safe while challenged.

This is the key for us to transform your mind, body, and life together. I want to meet your expectations. I must trust you and you must trust yourself to be able to do it. You also must trust that I have your best interests at heart. By the end of this book I hope I will have earned that trust with approachability, honesty, expertise, and results.

If I were to meet you right now, our interaction would go something like this:

"My name is Rupa. What's your name?"

"It's nice to meet you. Any injuries I should know about?"

"I'll say your name a lot in class. Don't think I'm picking on you; it comes from a good place—I promise."

"If you start shaking a little during class and feel a burn, that's normal."

"Take breaks if you need to, but I trust you came here to work hard, so make sure you are committed to form. And if you do take breaks, be sure that they are well-deserved and you make a quick comeback."

I start every interaction with a client that way because I know that names matter and that *you* matter. Our dynamic matters. If you've generously chosen to spend your valuable time, money, and effort with me, our time together must be comfortable, safe, efficient, and effective.

If we've established the fundamental groundwork of trust and support between us, I'd like you to think of this chapter as not merely an overview of how the Nalini Method works, but as an integral part of the entire workout. The Nalini Method fundamentals are not just about the equipment you do or do not need or about finding the time to exercise. They are about embracing the essence and heart of this book—the written equivalent of how I assertively and passionately teach my classes. I teach with the crucial belief that it is necessary to embrace the following tools, in order to become your own best teacher and build a successful workout.

The Basics

The basics are all those tiny things that can make a huge difference. Don't take them for granted. This is where you're setting yourself up—for success!

EQUIPMENT

All you need is your mood and your yoga mat!

Actually, all you need is this book, your mood, and your mat (or a towel or other supported surface, like a carpeted floor). In my studio, you will find a lot of props like blocks, weights, ankle weights, straps, and a barre. For this book, however, I've deliberately kept the workouts prop-free so as to simplify everything for you—while, of course, maintaining the challenge. I want you to be able to do these workouts easily anywhere and anytime. Whether you're at home, working out of town on a business trip, or even on vacation, these workouts can all be taken to go.

Last but certainly not least: the most important piece of equipment for all of these workouts is your *mindset*. In order for this book to be effective I need you to honestly acknowledge your mood, to state it, and to *own* it. I trust you to patiently search for your mood and name it as accurately as possible. When you do, you'll realize that you are truly built to last. You'll also enjoy the fruits of becoming your own best teacher harnessing seven powerful mind/body tools.

DRESS

It's best to do each workout barefoot, in clothing that makes you feel good and allows for a full range of motion. This workout is for you, by you, and about you, and I want you to feel good inside and out. (Choose your colors wisely!)

SPACE

Create a motivating atmosphere for yourself. Whether it be a sacred place in your home, on the patio, at a public park, or a spacious area in your hotel room, be conscious of where you choose to unfold your mat and mood. Keep the room warm, not cold or hot. A comfortable temperature will help your muscles move better.

TIME

I have shortened the length of my typical workout from one hour to about twenty to twenty-five minutes. This makes the seven workouts even easier to fit into your daily schedule.

Don't fret. This is still a transformative, total body workout! You will feel a full and complete challenge in this abbreviated, strategic time frame. Note that in the learning process, these workouts may take much longer. But as you become familiar with and master them, you will need less time to complete them.

The ultimate goal is to make all seven workouts a regular part of your daily life. They will serve as seven tools that can play a vital role in helping to manage your mood and create a stronger core, emotionally and physically.

You can use these workouts as your primary daily workout or as a supplement to your regular workout. Some of my clients only work out using the Nalini Method, and some like to switch it up and add my classes on the days they're not going to spin class, playing tennis, or running. The Nalini Method is flexible and rewarding enough to stand alone or be done alongside other fun activities. The workouts provide exceptional awareness and significant mind and body strength. You will find that not only will you have a stronger body, but also your moods will be greatly improved and manageable. Benefits like that can be needed and are accessible anytime. Thoughtfully plan for where and when you can consistently incorporate these workouts into your day and life. The more you do the workouts, the more muscle memory you'll develop emotionally and physically, and the seven workouts will soon become second nature. I strongly suggest you practice the Nalini Method a minimum of three times a week and up to seven times a week, depending, of course, on your moods!

FEEDBACK LOOP

Whether you are new to exercise and the Nalini Method, an experienced exerciser, or a current client, form is key. I see proper form and technique as a feedback loop. A positive feedback loop will occur when, armed with the detailed breakdowns in Part II, you are in charge. You monitor and hold yourself accountable to your form, intention, attitude, and breathing. When you do these things, they actually come back to heighten your form and the effectiveness of the workout. As your ability to give yourself feedback increases, so does your strength. As your strength increases, so does your ability to process more feedback. In time, your confidence in yourself and the routine increases.

A negative feedback loop will occur if you are armed with these detailed breakdowns but do not believe that you, no matter what your fitness level, are responsible for constantly checking in on your form. As a result, you will be led down a road of frustration with yourself, the workout, and me, causing your strength and ability to process any feedback to decrease. In time, your confidence in yourself and the routine will decrease.

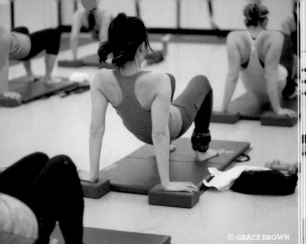
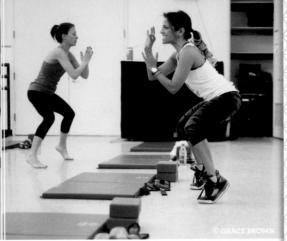

You must be willing to work through the exercises and be patient with yourself, whether you need to take breaks or simply adjust your form. Being in form means you are always thinking about form! When you are form-driven, you will feel that sense of firmness, strength, and muscle isolation in all your exercises, the proper release in your stretches, and mindfulness during the entire workout (because you don't have time to think of anything else).

Embrace the feedback loop. Without it, you cheat yourself out of the optimal workout.

How to Use This Book

There are three phases to each mood workout: *Pre-Workout*, *Workout*, and *Post-Workout*. Just as you ideally wouldn't show up to a class late or leave early, don't skip out on the Pre- and Post-Workouts; all three phases are equally important. Let's take a look here at the structured breakdown and how the Nalini Method works.

PHASE 1: THE PRE-WORKOUT

This part of the workout sets the tone for the rest of the session, so you must be mindful. Just before your workout, you'll be evaluating your mind and your body, asking yourself how you feel and acknowledging your mood. In each of the mood chapters, the Pre-Workout has the following four steps to get you prepared for an optimal, personalized session:

1 **I Am Feeling:**
Each chapter has an extensive list of synonyms for the given mood. See which words best match your mood, choosing from the lists or adding your own words. You'll notice that for some moods, certain words are listed twice; the word "frustrated" is seen in both the Anxiety and Doubt workouts, as "frustrated" relates to more than just one

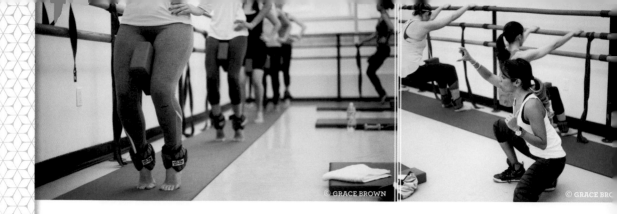
© GRACE BROWN   © GRACE BRO

mood. Remember this is about *you*. There is no right or wrong mood. This is not a test; it's a safe place. It's just you and your mat, so be honest and allow yourself to choose the best workout for your mood. If you're angry or anxious or chill, so be it. *It's all good.*

2 My Current Mood Is:

Write down your mood or say it out loud—and embrace it. Acknowledging your mood is the first step to *truly* managing it. Taking that extra moment not only to be aware of your mood but to name it allows you to eventually tame it. If you know it, you can own it!

3 My Emotional Weight Is:

You already learned about emotional versus physical weight and the emotional scale in Chapter 1. This is the time to measure your emotional weight. Don't judge the answer or overanalyze it. Simply choose among light, neutral, and heavy on the 1–10 emotional scale.

4 My Physical Symptoms Are:

You'll find a physical symptom list in each mood chapter. Determine which ones could be the physical manifestation of your mood. As with the emotionally driven synonyms and choosing your mood earlier, see if your physical symptoms match what's on the list to help you choose the most appropriate workout.

TEN COMMON **MOOD** THOUGHTS

The more clients I meet and talk to, the more I realize we're all so similar, going through the very same moods throughout the day. You'll find this sidebar in each mood chapter, where I list the most common thoughts associated with that mood that I've had or have heard—and that you've probably had, too! Relating to or not being able to relate to them will help guide you to choosing your best workout.

PHASE 2: THE WORKOUT

After choosing the mood that best suits you, you're ready to work out! You have to get your mind *and* body moving; both parts are crucial to the optimal workout. The Workout sections are as follows:

1 The Mantra

Each mood workout has a specific *mantra*: a quote or saying that acts as that mood's motto. The mantra is the new inspirational song to add to your playlist and listen to when you're in that mood. To truly appreciate and reap the benefits of every mood mantra, I've chosen to share my personal and sometimes challenging journeys in understanding each mantra myself. These mantras are life lessons I grew up with, based on sayings that my mom, Nalini, and my dad, Pinak, repeated often over the years. They did so in the hopes that if I could embrace them, I could live a happier and more vibrant life. They have not all come easily to me or to my students, but they are tools that, when fully learned and used continuously, can help manage your emotional weight. Over time, these mantras will naturally become part of your playlist and allow you to successfully understand, approach, and manage your mood.

2 How to Use the Mantra

Be patient when learning the mantras. Not only will you grow to better understand and appreciate them, but they will allow you to manage your thoughts and feelings instead of them managing you. Over time, as you explore the mantras and deal with your mood, which will sometimes feel like a mountain to climb, the mantras will empower your journey and become a part of you. They *stick*.

Through my own life and teaching experiences, I have found repetition is key. It's not that we are not smart enough and can't get it the first time. It's that we need to constantly practice and hold ourselves accountable to really embrace and live out the benefits of what we are learning. "Practice makes perfect" is really true!

Think of yourself as the train in *The Little Engine That Could* by Watty Piper. The book's mantra, "I think I can—I think I can—I think I can," resonated when the book was published in 1930, and continues to resonate with every generation that reads it. Those simple and encouraging words carried so much power, allowing the little engine to eventually believe it could overcome the seemingly impossible task of travelling over a big mountain, a goal usually reserved for larger engines. Other than the valuable lesson of the power of a mental playlist, the story also demonstrates that when you commit to and repeat simple words of wisdom over time, they become a common, healthy

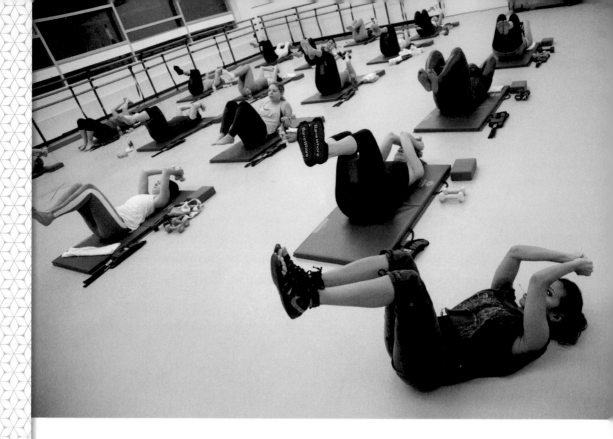

part of you and enable you to chip away at emotional weight and eventually accomplish your goals. You are fully capable of tapping into that *I think I can—I think I can—I think I can* mentality again! Use the simple words of the mantras as a loving, hands-on support system. They are there unconditionally to keep you going.

Some of you may enjoy reading the mantra story every time you work out; some of you may read it every once in a while. Some of you may really relate to my stories; some of you may feel inspired to come up with your own mantra and story, one uniquely tailored to your own experiences. I encourage you to, as it will then resonate as powerfully for you as mine do for me. You'll be amazed at how quickly these mantras can help you on and off the mat, during your workout and in all aspects of your daily life.

3 Why This Workout

In this section, I share with you how the chosen mantras and exercises will channel your mood. If all the moods could manifest into a physical flow and the meaning behind the mantras could morph into exercises, that would be the workouts themselves!

I wanted the moods and mantras to come to physical life, so each routine is very different. And because each mood is different, each workout has a different vibe. For example, in Chapter 5: The Stress Workout, the mantra is "Shut up. Sit. Smile." When you're very stressed-out, shutting up, sitting, and smiling could be the last thing on your mind and can be incredibly difficult. And, if you do in fact calm down, it's usually some form of support that gets you there. So I deliberately designed the Stress workout to be very calming and to use the wall as "support" in every exercise. Once you embrace the carefully selected mantras, they will help you with enhanced purpose and drive to focus in and effectively complete the exercises and channel your mood.

4 My Workout Intention (Emotional or Physical) Is:

Here, you will state your intention, what you hope to gain or accomplish from working out, by writing it down, thinking it, *or* saying it out loud. This will allow you to have clarity and prepare your mind and body for a successful workout. Whether you're doing one of my workouts or running in the park, it's always nice to have an intention, a reason to motivate yourself and to remind yourself of why you're doing what you're doing. Perhaps it's as simple as "I want to fully commit to the mantra," or "I just need to do this, it makes me feel better," or you have a physical goal in mind, or maybe you've chosen to reflect on a person or situation that could use a bit of extra love. While I'm working out, whenever I feel my motivation flagging, I remind myself of my intention and it really encourages me to stay committed and keep pushing.

Whether you've had the worst or best possible day, when you set a personal intention, you are forced to ask yourself what is important to you. Reflecting on "What is my goal, and what do I want to get out of this workout?" will make your workout that much more effective.

Your intention can change with each workout. Sometimes you'll have a purely physical goal, and other times you'll want to concentrate on a more emotionally related intention. Either way, choose one that specifically relates to your mood of the moment—something that your mood needs or craves as reinforcement.

Remember: anything you think or say is totally fine. There are no judgments. Just own your intention! It's *yours*.

These are some intention examples I've had myself and heard from clients. As you'll see, anything counts:

- I am going to tap into my breath.

- I will really use the mantra today as something steady to come back to.

- I need to do this workout. My intention is to be open to figuring out why I need it. I just know I do.

- I want to enjoy my body throughout the duration of this workout.

- I want to challenge and push myself.

- I am so stressed, I will start screaming if I don't do a lot of crunches.

- My intention is to commit to my posture.

- I will finish this workout even if I don't want to.

- After what I've been through, I will remember that being able to move is a gift.

- My intention is to feel a lot better when this workout is over.

- I may be on the verge of tears, but I will be patient and do this for myself.

- Even if I take breaks, I will not take a break during the Plank.

- I'm really tired today so if I quit halfway through, I am not going to beat myself up. I know I'll do better next time.

- My boss was so awful at work today that I am ready to throttle him, so I need to get this anger out. I'm going to channel that negative energy into the fiercest workout possible!

- I am full of energy but it's all over the place, so my intention is to focus right now.

MUSIC

Nothing gets the blood flowing more quickly than a song you love. It could be the beat, the lyrics, or the message—we all have music that motivates us to keep on moving.

I've included some of my favorite songs from different decades, in different genres. From one-hit wonders to classics, each of these songs encourages you to explore the mood in question. They also allow you to engage with each specific mood and tie into the mantra.

Have fun choosing songs that work for you. It's a great way to identify and embrace the many positive and negative sides of your mood.

5 The Exercises

Read the exercises first, before you try them. Each exercise has been broken down very clearly, and in a specific order, so you can easily do them and watch your form naturally fall into place. The transitions make it even easier for you to get that flow going as you move seamlessly from one exercise to the next. (Note: each exercise chapter has an intro page with all the exercises in order, along with a small photo. This will become a "refer to" page once a Workout is memorized.)

Bear in mind that, like any new skill, these exercises will not be mastered immediately. If you are new to exercise routines or if you haven't worked out in a while, take a look at the photographs. Stand in front of a mirror and mimic the poses until you know you resemble what I'm demonstrating in each shot. Are your muscles engaged properly? Do you feel the target of the exercise? You don't want to follow just to follow. I want you to train yourself to move with confidence, purpose, and intention. Tap into your internal athlete, practice the exercises, and strive to get better at isolating the targeted muscles and intentions more effectively each time.

I always say the most advanced student is the one who is consistently monitoring their form and engaged in the feedback loop. In my classes, this is the true sign of strength. Coming back to questions like "Am I pulling in my abdominals?" or "Am I in form and following the right count?" will keep your Workout that much more results driven and fulfilling. I am passionate about form, and if you need to take breaks, so be it. Just remember to make sure they are well deserved! Be form driven!

While you're in the learning process, it's more important to complete the whole routine. This allows you to figure out what to do better next time. Believe me, it will get easier, and a lot faster than you think. Your muscles will know what to do, your ability to "teach" yourself and guide yourself back to proper alignment will increase, and the mantras will become a welcome part of your life.

You will get the best results by executing constant feedback. At any fitness level, always make tiny adjustments and take advantage of the nuances and notes written into these exercises so you can continually fine-tune your Workout. Before you know it, you'll be choosing your Workouts with confidence and transitioning seamlessly through each exercise.

HOW THE COUNT WORKS

Every exercise has a section called "Series," which gives you instructions on how many reps and which movements to do for each exercise. Every movement is connected to a count. The count is as important as form, and one of your goals with the Nalini Method is to master it. There are several different counts:

- **Single:** The single count is what you'd expect. It's a simple up/down (or applicable variations like down/up, out/in, open/close) motion. You will move an inch up or down (or in the given direction). You should be precise and focused with every rep.

- **Double:** The double count breaks the single count into parts. Instead of up/down, you'll move up-up/down-down. It's a four-part motion, and instead of moving fluidly, you're treating each part as its own individual precise motion.

- **Pulses:** Think of a pulse as a bounce, a quick repeated beat. It's the quickest of the counts. Once you're in the most intense part of the exercise (for example, the lowest point of your squat), instead of going fully up or down, you do a repeated tiny pulsing motion while you stay in position.

- **Multi:** This is definitely the most complicated of the counts. It is a combination of a pulse and a hold. This count consists of three pulses and a drop, specifically. For example: up-up-up/down or lift-lift-lift/lower. The drop is usually a deep drop, meaning you feel a full range. For example, in pelvic tucks you would pulse at your highest point three times, then drop to your lowest point as the down motion.

- **Hold:** This is where you remain stationary, holding on to particular muscles while focusing intently on form. This can sometimes be harder than any contraction or movement. You will be holding your form steady in the most challenging part of the exercise, like in the deepest part of your squat or the highest part of your abdominal crunch. Do the holds in full; although it's tempting to move, perform your holds for at least the count of five. They are there for a reason!

So how will this apply to your workout? Take push-ups. Instead of twenty straight push-ups, we may do ten double count and ten single count. Instead of twenty sit-ups, there may be fifteen multi counts and a five count hold at the end. These counts are a great way to add variety and new challenges to your workouts. Once you're familiar with these different tempos, you'll notice a huge difference and will really own your workout. That's the beauty of it: every second of your workout is accounted for and every workout will be different, even if some of the exercises stay the same! To make the counts easier and find workout videos, visit my website: www.nalinimethod.com.

Important Workout Tips

POSTURE

How you stand is how you feel.

Standing tall, with your chest up, and being conscious of your eye focus with a sense of confidence and purpose translates to a better mood. Standing carelessly or slumping while waiting for direction, drive, or courage translates to a weaker mood. In other words, your posture is the physical manifestation of your emotional weight.

The benefit of standing upright is building smart muscles that help you stay open. Even more profound are the mind/emotional and mood-related benefits of good posture. When you stand tall, your life is broader and the sky is the limit. I'm not kidding. That extra inch physically is an extra mile mentally.

Every workout begins with some form of meditation/focusing exercise where I want you to stand tall physically and emotionally. Even if some of the exercises aren't done when you're upright, you should still be aware of your postural energy. Make this a habit. If you commit to your posture during the workout, you will start to see that habit follow you outside your Nalini Method time. You'll soon see yourself sitting taller in the car, standing taller at meetings, and feeling more confident in general.

STRETCHING

Nearly all of the stretches in the workouts are placed strategically after an exercise that targets the same muscles. You'll strengthen and then immediately lengthen the same area. It's important to be aware of this dichotomy to tap into an efficient use of your focus and time.

What makes the actual stretch effective? For me, I need to feel that my body is going in two opposite directions, as if it were a rubber band. Those opposite directions are best when linked to an inhale and an exhale. This opposition makes you feel the stretch more, and that little internal tug-of-war (push and pull) creates the space to feel the stretch.

Rather than just holding a stretch and waiting for something to happen, remember that every movement and second count. Each stretch shouldn't be thought of as a rest stop or something to do mindlessly. Tapping into that resistance between two body parts—with an inhale moving one part one way and an exhale moving another part the opposite way—creates that special yin and yang, and makes you effectively feel the stretch. Concentrate on your breathing, connect it to the oppositional pull, and make it challenging. Last, don't get caught up in the "look" of flexibility; instead, embrace creating the resistance needed to feel the stretch properly.

Stretches are like the light at the end of the tunnel: you'll work hard, look forward to them, and feel like you deserve that release. Enjoy it.

BREATHING

Think of your breath as your life force. When you're doing a stretch, in particular, your inhale and exhale will bring life to those areas that feel tight. Think about the muscles you are engaging and imagine your breath flowing into them. Try to use your breathing as a way to relax your mind and encourage your body to feel alive.

Breathing is a terrific way to become present really quickly. When you focus on your breath you are more connected to the actual moment and you breathe new life into your mind that has otherwise been consumed by your mood. It's literally and figuratively a breath of fresh air for your thoughts and thought patterns.

All you need to think about with the Nalini Method is that each breath is long, full, and intentional. You'll know a breath is full when you feel an inflation and deflation within your body—and you can then connect it to a smarter movement that reflects your chosen pace.

Common Exercises

You'll notice that certain exercises are repeated throughout the seven workouts:

Meditative Poses: These will come in different forms (such as standing, kneeling, or stretching) but they all help reinforce your intention and the chapter's mantra, and enable you to become fully present and focused.

Down Dog: I love Down Dog as a stand-alone stretch and a transitional pose between exercises. So strike that balance, keep it active, and yet maintain its intention of relaxing and replenishing the body.

Child's Pose: These are sprinkled in strategically, usually after a super-challenging series. The intention here is that you worked hard, so now you get to chill hard. Enjoy every second of this pose.

Push-Ups: Most women want to do bent-leg Push-Ups, but with the Nalini Method you will always be doing straight-leg Push-Ups. My clients will tell you, even if they come to a class after just having a baby, they're going to be doing straight-leg Push-Ups. Embrace this! I know you are strong enough, or will quickly become strong enough. Even if it is a micro-bend of your elbows, the smallest Push-Up in the world, it counts in my eyes. It's totally fine at first to do two with perfect form, take a break, make a quick comeback, do five in form, and continue until you finish the series. They all count. You will be astonished at how quickly your muscles respond. I love seeing the pride on a newbie's face when he or she can effortlessly pull off a Push-Up sequence for the first time.

Plank: The Plank is an exercise commonly used in many different forms and workouts, as it is highly effective and efficient. You're using your body's own weight to build muscle and core strength. Like Push-Ups, you will see results rather quickly the more you do the Plank. If they seem impossible, aim and structure a hold time that works for you. For example, try for at least a ten-second hold, and then work up to the count indicated. Feel successful that you did the ten-second hold, since that is what you said you'd do. As always, it's okay to take breaks so long as you recover quickly and keep your head in the game. Feel free to structure your breaks (e.g., ten-second increments in Plank), which may make you feel more empowered.

PHASE 3: THE POST-WORKOUT

You made it! You've completed a true mind/body workout, and it's time to evaluate its effectiveness. The Post-Workout recap is as important as you owning your mood, setting your intention, saying the mantra, and doing the exercises. Awareness, as you know, is empowerment. Just as you've made yourself aware Pre-Workout, it's as crucial to acknowledge where you are Post-Workout. Always do the following:

1 Post-Workout Recap

At the end of each workout, you should feel effects immediately. You are in a new moment—so time to embrace it! Has your mood shifted? Has your emotional weight changed? Is your physical body feeling stronger/better?

2 My Post-Workout Mood Is:

Own your mood now! Write it down, think it, or say it out loud. Maybe your mood has heightened; maybe you have new tools to tackle it; maybe it has completely changed. However you feel, be present, appreciate a sense of completion and respect where you find yourself emotionally and physically.

Now, we're really ready. Let's get the party started!

PART II
THE MIND/BODY ROUTINES

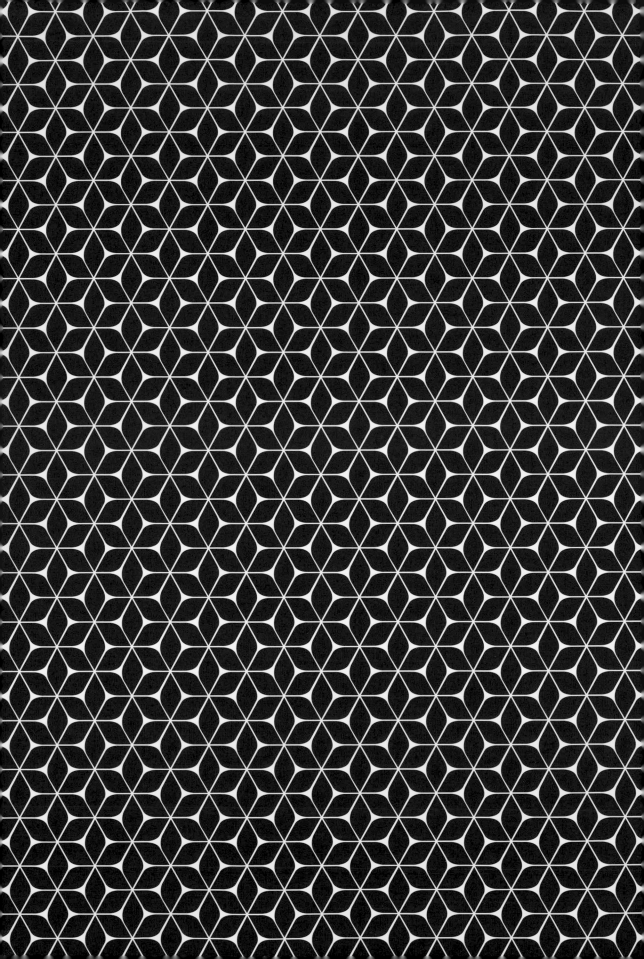

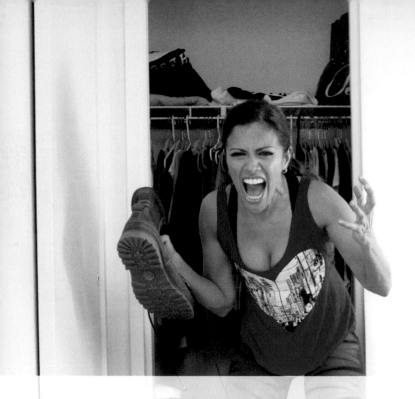

— CHAPTER 3 —

THE ANGER WORKOUT

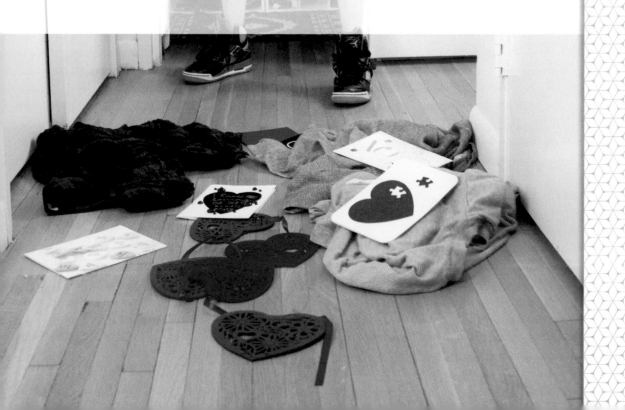

THE ANGER EXERCISES

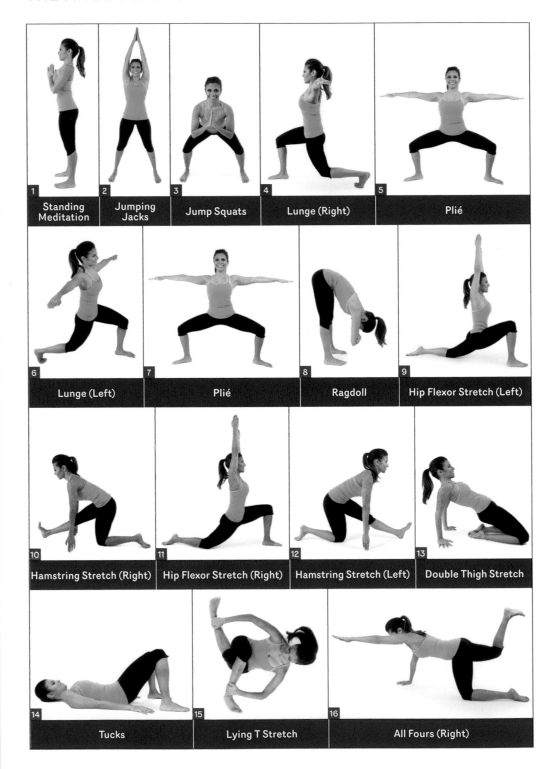

1. Standing Meditation
2. Jumping Jacks
3. Jump Squats
4. Lunge (Right)
5. Plié
6. Lunge (Left)
7. Plié
8. Ragdoll
9. Hip Flexor Stretch (Left)
10. Hamstring Stretch (Right)
11. Hip Flexor Stretch (Right)
12. Hamstring Stretch (Left)
13. Double Thigh Stretch
14. Tucks
15. Lying T Stretch
16. All Fours (Right)

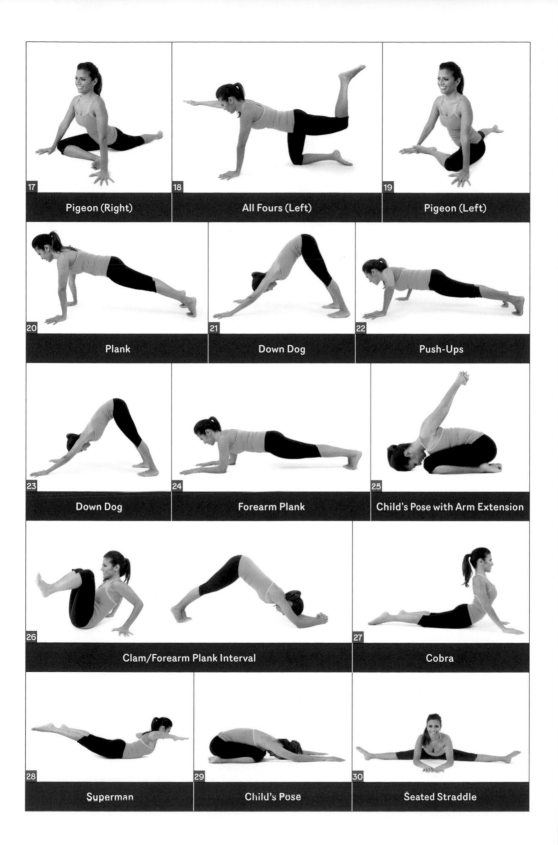

17 Pigeon (Right)

18 All Fours (Left)

19 Pigeon (Left)

20 Plank

21 Down Dog

22 Push-Ups

23 Down Dog

24 Forearm Plank

25 Child's Pose with Arm Extension

26 Clam/Forearm Plank Interval

27 Cobra

28 Superman

29 Child's Pose

30 Seated Straddle

Anger is a mood that can seep into every pore of your body and weigh on you so much that you feel you could just burst from the pressure. Often, you're angry about being angry! Anger has a unique way of getting you to commit to black-and-white thinking so fast that your flexible mind gets left in the dust.

Ask yourself this: What is that one rigid angry thought you keep coming back to? The thought that makes you feel red all over? The thought that is making you want to start a protest, run around in circles, kick some butt, or explode? What thought is stuck on replay? That is the thought I want you to own.

What is the emotional weight of that thought and its resulting mood, and how is it manifesting in your physical body?

THE PRE-WORKOUT

1 **I Am Feeling:**

- ☐ Angry
- ☐ Annoyed
- ☐ Antagonistic
- ☐ Bitter
- ☐ Crabby
- ☐ Cranky
- ☐ Disgruntled
- ☐ Envious
- ☐ Exasperated
- ☐ Frustrated
- ☐ Furious
- ☐ Grouchy

- ☐ Heightened Defenses (Fight or Flight)
- ☐ Hotheaded
- ☐ Incensed
- ☐ Indignant
- ☐ Irritated
- ☐ Jealous
- ☐ Mad
- ☐ Mean
- ☐ Mopey
- ☐ Morose
- ☐ Petulant

- ☐ Provoking
- ☐ Quarrelsome
- ☐ Raging
- ☐ Resentful
- ☐ Riled-Up
- ☐ Seething
- ☐ Stormy
- ☐ Sulky
- ☐ Touchy
- ☐ Vengeful
- ☐ Venting
- ☐ Wrathful

Choose from the list above, or add your own words. Then write down your mood *or* say it out loud and embrace it.

2 **My Current Mood Is:**

_____

3 My Emotional Weight Is:

```
1                        5                        10
Light                 Neutral                   Heavy
```

4 My Physical Symptoms Are:

- ☐ Adrenaline Rush
- ☐ Aggression
- ☐ Clenching
- ☐ Cramps
- ☐ Crying
- ☐ Cursing
- ☐ Feeling Flushed
- ☐ Fist Pounding

- ☐ Goosebumps
- ☐ Head Rubbing
- ☐ Heat Flashes
- ☐ Heavy Breathing
- ☐ Heavy Chest
- ☐ Jaw Clenching
- ☐ Pacing
- ☐ Prickly Sensations

- ☐ Raised Voice
- ☐ Rapid Heartbeat
- ☐ Shaking
- ☐ Stomachache
- ☐ Sweating
- ☐ Teeth Grinding
- ☐ Tightness

TEN COMMON ANGRY THOUGHTS

- I can't believe my boyfriend disrespected me like that. I will never forget what he did.
- I had a fight with my brother. When will he ever understand?
- My son's teacher ignored the kid who was bullying my son, and *he* got in trouble instead of the bully.
- That rotten driver nearly hit my car. It was my right-of-way!
- I worked for weeks on a presentation at work and my jealous coworker took all the credit for it.
- I took a whole day off of work to let the cable guy in and he never showed.
- My husband promised to do something really important and surprise, surprise . . . he forgot.
- It's simple. Everyone is stupid.
- Ugh . . . I know it may be a tiny amount, but I still got ripped off.
- After all I've done for our friendship, she has the nerve to reverse it and get mad at me!

THE WORKOUT

1 Mantra for Anger:

The solution is born before the problem.

I used to be afraid of anger. My traditional Indian upbringing convinced me that anger should be avoided at all costs, as it would harm me. One quote from Buddha about anger has always summed it up for me: "Holding on to anger is like drinking poison and expecting the other person to die." Wow! Bottom line: anger is scary and powerful. It was only recently that I opened myself up to the power of anger. And boy, did I open myself up!

As a result, I've experienced the danger of unmanaged anger as well as the amazing potential of anger managed properly. What I've learned is that anger comes in many forms and coping with it comes in many forms as well. The key is to understand how anger uniquely manifests in your mind, body, and life, and how to manage it in a way that solicits results that can transform your anger into drive, passion, and action.

Quite simply, I find that most people, myself included, get angry because of some sort of problem they see, feel, and experience.

What if I told you that the world was not filled with problems? You might think I was idealistic, unaware, and unrealistic—exactly what I thought about my ever-so-calm dad when I was growing up. You failed a test? According to him, this was not a problem. You broke your leg? Not a problem. You have a deadly virus? Not a problem. As a kid, I was dumbfounded. How were these not legitimate problems? They sure felt like problems to *me*. Besides, everyone around me, from friends to doctors, also defined them that way.

My dad's favorite mantra has always been "The solution is born before the problem." I heard him say it nearly every day growing up. When I finally understood the power it has to transform one's anger, it became my favorite saying, too.

Thinking of a problem as a situation that is unwelcome or harmful can be limiting and distracting. When we attach ourselves to dissecting and focusing on the negativity of the problem, we take away valuable time and effort from finding the solution. When we allow our problem to emotionally outweigh our search for a solution, we aren't as open to the many possible solutions. In fact, both solutions and problems are just options—except one works and the other doesn't.

This rang true for me in 2008, when I was looking to expand my business. I confidently, yet nervously, wrote to the CEO of a large and extremely successful company that I thought would be a terrific fit for my teaching. Much to my surprise, he wrote back the same day! The following week, representatives of the company came to take my class and see the studio. I was revelling in energy and enthusiasm as we met and talked about a potential partnership. Although nothing was solidified, the possibility gave me something to work on and look forward to.

As I was daydreaming about a buyout, in reality things were slowing down. I wrote a follow-up email and didn't get a reply. I waited and waited, and was starting to get angry because I felt abandoned and disrespected. When they finally contacted me two months later, I was very relieved. They brought more people to the studio. Once again, there was momentum. We discussed the possibility of partnering as well as building a custom space in their new facility, which was set to open in three months. They said I could expect a formal proposal in two weeks and the final transaction in four. I left the meeting on cloud nine. After working so passionately to build my small business, I couldn't imagine a better situation; everything from the timing to the deal itself seemed perfect.

Nothing arrived. I followed up again and again—and nothing. The company's employees would come to my class and mention overhearing something about an expansion but still, no communication from the big guys. I felt abandoned again. Why were they treating me this way? Why couldn't they just say yes or no instead of dragging this out? I had been so excited and my dream had seemed so close. Why was I feeling like I was being punished?

Oh, I was *angry*, all right. Was this merely cavalier treatment or was this truly how the business world operated and I just needed to get used to it? All of this was new to me and I was a mess. I felt defensive. I wanted to write a list of all my top qualities and why the world was a better place with me in it and holler it from the rooftops. Yet, I also wanted to crawl into a hole, to cry, scream, and lick my wounds from insecurity. My tension was so off the charts I needed to get a retainer from my dentist to stop me from grinding my teeth.

I should have been following my dad's advice, right? By allowing this company's unresponsiveness to become the problem, I was falling into the trap of believing that their offer was the only way to achieve my goals. I was focusing all my energy on trying to "fix" things and make contact with the company.

Once I realized this, I chose to see the situation through my dad's eyes. According to him, when something isn't working out the way you planned or hoped, it's easy to forget your original goals and intentions. He flips things around so, in his mind, what some call a problem is actually a solution that simply isn't working. The turning point happens when you remember what you set out to do in the beginning and realize you once thought of your current problem as a solution. With this business situation, my original goal had been to add new meaning to my work and life. When I stopped fuming, I could see that selling my business to a larger company was *only one way* to accomplish my goals. There would *always* be many more ways to reach my goals.

Over the years, I have found my dad's mantra to be invaluable. You can also see that "The solution is born before the problem" because we seek out solutions for future problems all the time. From buying insurance on a new phone, to carrying an umbrella for a rainy day, to writing a will, to accepting the death of a loved one, we are constantly thinking of potential solutions for problems we could face in our lives. But when we forget this mantra, we often get angry and consumed by the problem and fail to discover and revel in a world filled with infinite solutions.

Truly embracing this mantra has given me a lively openness to and active acceptance of anger. It has transformed how I deal with problems that used to send me right into a rage. Like everyone, I still get angry, but I now have the tools to quickly and resolutely bounce back, avoiding a prolonged attachment to the emotional weight of the anger that can pull me down. Thanks to my dad's mantra, my life feels consistently hopeful and my true self is calmer. I always know, no matter what the circumstance, that "The solution is born before the problem." I just have to look for it and I'll find it.

Instead of my anger/problem weighing me down, I can now use it as a starting point to lift me up toward a healthy solution.

2 How to Use the Mantra

When you're really angry, all you can do is focus on the rage, right? It's hard to imagine nurturing your anger to a place where the edge can be taken off and a solution can be born.

But it can happen. Take all that energy that's focused on the problem/source of your anger and refocus it on discovering a solution/outlet for your anger. Focus on the burning feeling inside and use it as fuel to transform your anger into a productive session burning with possibilities.

Take a lesson from my dad, and think of your problem—your anger—as a solution that doesn't work. The true solution is the option that *does* work.

Solutions come in all shapes and sizes. It could be as simple as suddenly letting it all go in the blink of an eye, or as hard as committing to changing your environment entirely. Or, your solution may come from somewhere surprising, like prayer, time passing, or reflecting on an angry moment from your past that no longer makes you mad. It may not be pretty, ideal, or perfect, but lightening the emotional burden of your anger even a little bit will allow you to inch your way toward a solution that is ultimately better for you emotionally and physically.

Repeat "The solution is born before the problem" to yourself and commit to a kick-ass workout.

3 Why the Anger Workout

By now you have taken the time to reflect on what is causing you to go from zero to one hundred in less than a second, and how that source weighs on you emotionally and physically.

The flow of this exercise series is designed for you to tap into the excess adrenaline of your anger and channel that energy into fast-moving and challenging exercises. This workout is all about the burn and being effective. When you're angry you don't want to waste a second of your time—you need an outlet. That is why this workout has more exercises than any of the other workouts in the book, so bring your anger on!

Embrace your mood, reflect on the mantra, and let it provide you with all the drive necessary to find a solution and make it through this rep-filled routine.

4 My Anger Workout Intention (Emotional or Physical) Is:

(Write down, think, or say out loud.)

MUSIC

Choose music that makes your mood feel supported. Here are a few suggestions that can help you feel understood and get that aggression out!

1960s: "Paint It Black" ▪ The Rolling Stones

1970s: "Locomotive Breath" ▪ Jethro Tull

1980s: "Tainted Love" ▪ Soft Cell

1990s: "You Oughta Know" ▪ Alanis Morissette

2000s: "Break Stuff" ▪ Limp Bizkit

2010s: "Beautiful Pain" ▪ Eminem

1. Standing Meditation

FOCUS: Total body awareness

MANTRA: The solution is born before the problem.

BREATHING TECHNIQUE: Inhale your chest up/Exhale your shoulders back.

GET IN POSITION: Begin by standing with your feet hip-width apart. Keep your feet parallel, with your toes in front of your heels. Maintain straight legs. Point your tailbone down. Tighten your abs by pulling your belly button in toward your spine. Stand tall as you lengthen your abs and chest up and away from your hips. Keep your chest open, with your shoulders back and down, away from your ears. Your head should be in line with your spine. Focus forward. Bring your palms together in front of your chest.

SERIES: 30-second hold or longer

NEED TO MODIFY? Close your eyes to help you focus better.

TRANSITION: Jump into exercise 2.

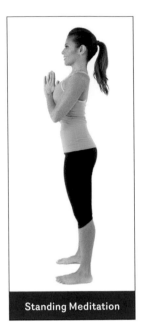

Standing Meditation

2. Jumping Jacks

FOCUS: Total body cardio

INTENTION: "I'm here. I'm ready. Let's do this."

GET IN POSITION: Begin by standing with your feet and legs together. Keep your feet parallel, with your toes in front of your heels. Point your tailbone down. Tighten your abs by pulling your belly button in toward your spine. Stand tall as you lengthen your abs and chest up and away from your hips. Keep your chest open, with your shoulders back and down, away from your ears. Your arms should be straight

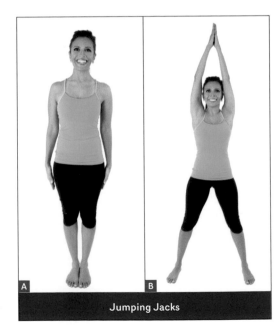

Jumping Jacks

down by your sides, palms facing in toward your body. Keep your head in line with your spine. Focus forward.

GET MOVING: Jump your feet out wider than your hips, lifting your arms toward the ceiling. Jump your feet back in, bringing your arms back down to your sides. Continue jumping your feet wider than your hips with your arms up and then your feet back together as your arms go down. Jump high, wide, and fast.

SERIES: 30 single count, *out/in*

LOOK OUT FOR: Moving too slowly. (The idea is to get the heart rate up!) Not jumping your feet wide enough. Being sloppy with your posture. (Jump with confidence!)

NEED TO MODIFY? Tender knees or back: Do Standing March (p. 169) instead.

TRANSITION: Keep your legs wide on the last jump and squat down; flow into exercise 3.

3. Jump Squats

FOCUS: Total body cardio

INTENTION: "I have power; it's up to me to use it."

GET IN POSITION: Begin by standing with your feet and knees wider than your hips. Keep your feet parallel, with your toes in front of your heels. Bend your knees and drop your hips. Continue to bend your knees directly over your heels, keeping them in line with your toes. (It should feel comfortable.) Try to lower your hips just far enough that they are in line with your knees. Lean your upper body forward at a 45-degree angle. Tighten your abs by pulling your belly button in toward your spine. Keep your chest open, with your shoulders back and down, away from your ears. Place your palms together in front of your chest. Your head should be in line with your spine. Focus forward.

GET MOVING: From your squat position, jump high enough that your toes spring off the floor while reaching your arms toward the ceiling. Land in a strong, supported squat with your knees at a 90-degree angle and palms

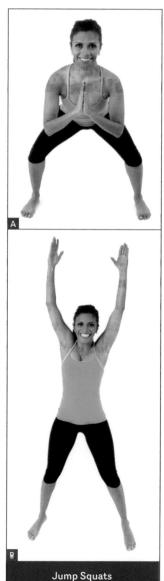

Jump Squats

together in front of your chest. Be mindful of your knees and back as you continue to jump up and down.

SERIES: 20 single count jumps *up/down* (After your last jump, stay in your squat and keep your feet flat on the floor for the remaining movements in the series.) 10 single count, *down/up* 10 pulses, *down/up* 10-second hold

LOOK OUT FOR: Not jumping high enough. Bringing your feet together upon landing versus maintaining a squat. Sinking your butt too low in the squat. (Be mindful of knee safety!)

NEED TO MODIFY? Tender knees or back: Skip the jumping and continue to squat down and up, following the same series.

TRANSITION: Turn your feet and your body to the right; flow into exercise 4.

4. Lunge (Right)

FOCUS: Thighs, glutes, and arms

INTENTION: "I'm increasing my emotional and physical strength."

GET IN POSITION: Begin with your feet hip-width apart, with your right foot about 2–3 feet in front of your left foot. Keep both of your feet parallel, with your toes in front of your heels. Raise your left heel off the floor. Bend both knees and drop your hips, forming a 90-degree angle with both legs. Tighten your abs by pulling your belly button in toward your spine. Lift your abs and chest up and away from your hips. Keep your chest open, with your shoulders back and down, away from your ears. Lift your arms up and across from your shoulders, forming a T-shape. Keep your palms facing down. Your head should be in line with your spine. Focus forward.

GET MOVING: Bend both of your knees as you lower your hips down and up. Pretend your back is sliding up and down an imaginary wall, as you lean back. Maintain a 90-degree angle with your right knee, keeping it in line with your right heel. Make sure your left heel is all the way up as you maintain a 90-degree angle with your left knee. Keep reaching through your fingertips as you lengthen your arms and keep them up and across from your shoulders.

SERIES: 5-second hold 10 single count, *down/up* 10 pulses, *down/down* 10-second hold

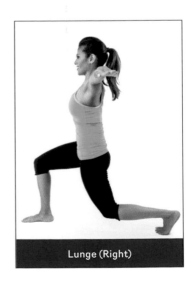

Lunge (Right)

LOOK OUT FOR: Leaning forward and not maintaining a flat back. Bending your front knee too far over your front foot. Not lifting your back heel high enough. Rounding your shoulders and chest. Not keeping your arms up and across from your shoulders.

NEED TO MODIFY? Tender knees: Keep your back leg straight and follow the same series.

TRANSITION: Turn your feet and your body counterclockwise to center; flow into exercise 5.

5. Plié

FOCUS: Inner thighs and glutes

INTENTION: "I have the power to be grounded."

GET IN POSITION: Begin with your feet wider than your hips. Turn both of your feet out to a 45-degree angle. (Think two o'clock and ten o'clock.) Bend your knees and drop your hips. Continue to bend your knees directly over your heels, keeping them in line with your toes. (It should feel comfortable.)

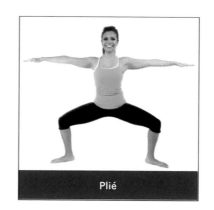

Plié

Try to lower your hips to the level of your knees. Keep your pelvis slightly tucked (as if you're straddling a horse). Tighten your abs by pulling your belly button in toward your spine. Lift your abs and chest up and away from your hips. Keep your chest open, with your shoulders back and down, away from your ears. Lift your arms up and across from your shoulders, forming a T-shape. Keep your palms facing down. Your head should be in line with your spine. Focus forward.

GET MOVING: Bend both of your knees as you lower your hips down and up. Pretend your back is sliding up and down an imaginary wall as you lean back. Keep your hips low and push your thighs and knees back to engage your inner thighs. Keep your stance wide with your knees in line with the direction of your toes. Keep reaching through your fingertips as you lengthen your arms and keep them up and across from your shoulders.

SERIES: 5-second hold 10 single count, *down/up* 10 pulses, *down/up* 10-second hold

LOOK OUT FOR: Leaning forward and not maintaining a flat back. Sticking your butt out. Rounding your shoulders and chest. Not keeping your arms up and across from your shoulders.

NEED TO MODIFY? Tender knees: Turn your feet in to decrease the turnout of your hips.

TRANSITION: Turn your feet and your body to the left; flow into exercise 6.

6. Lunge (Left)

Repeat exercise 4 with your left foot forward.

TRANSITION: Turn your feet and your body clockwise to center; flow into exercise 7.

7. Plié

Repeat exercise 5.

TRANSITION: Bend at your waist and fold your body over, walk your feet closer together, and flow into exercise 8.

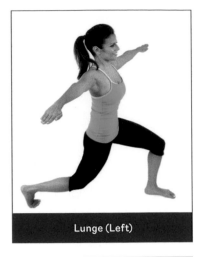

Lunge (Left)

8. Ragdoll

FOCUS: Hamstrings

BREATHING TECHNIQUE: Inhale your hips up/Exhale your upper body toward the floor.

GET IN POSITION: Begin by standing with your feet hip-width apart. Keep your feet parallel, with your toes in front of your heels. Reach your arms toward the floor as you fold your upper body over your legs, lengthening your spine. Grab hold of your elbows with your opposing hands. Maintain straight legs. (Soften your knees if your lower back or hamstrings are tight.) Hang, letting gravity pull your upper body toward the floor. Release any tension in your head and neck.

SERIES: 10-second hold

NEED TO MODIFY? Tight hamstrings or back: Keep your legs bent. (Don't pressure yourself to straighten your legs.)

TRANSITION: Step your left leg back; flow into exercise 9.

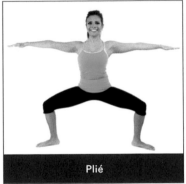

Plié

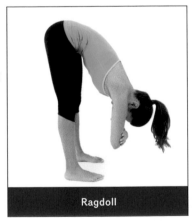

Ragdoll

9. Hip Flexor Stretch (Left)

FOCUS: Hip flexor

BREATHING TECHNIQUE: Inhale your left hip forward/Exhale your right hip back. Inhale your abs in and up/Exhale your upper body back.

GET IN POSITION: Begin with your right leg in front in a lunge position, with your right knee over your right heel. Keep your left leg parallel and on the ground, with your left foot in line with your left hip. Turn your left hip forward and make sure your hips are squared. Tuck your hips forward as you lift your abs and chest up and away from your hips. Reach your arms straight up toward the ceiling. Keep your palms facing in. Tighten your abs by pulling your belly button in toward your spine. Lean your upper body back. Keep your chest open, with your shoulders back and down, away from your ears. Your head should be in line with your spine. Focus forward.

SERIES: 10-second hold

NEED TO MODIFY? Tight hips: Keep your hands on the floor on either side of your front foot.

TRANSITION: Shift your weight back and straighten your right leg; flow into exercise 10.

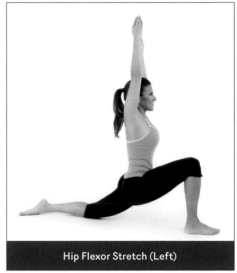

Hip Flexor Stretch (Left)

10. Hamstring Stretch (Right)

FOCUS: Hamstring, back, and IT band

BREATHING TECHNIQUE: Inhale and dig your right heel down into the floor/Exhale and reach your hips back. Inhale your right hip back/Exhale your left hip in. Inhale your chest forward/Exhale your shoulders back and down.

GET IN POSITION: Begin on your left knee with your right leg extended in front of you. Flex your right foot and press your right heel firmly into the floor. Turn your left hip

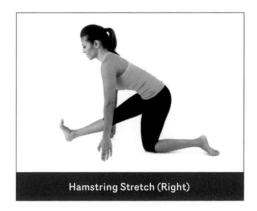

Hamstring Stretch (Right)

forward and make sure your hips are squared. Keep your back left leg at a 90-degree angle. Keep your left foot in line with your left knee. Keep your arms straight by your sides with your palms facing in and lean forward with a flat back. (Don't feel the need to do a split or touch the floor fully with your hands.) Your arms should help you maintain balance. (Not touching or barely touching the floor is fine!) Keep your right leg straight with your knee up toward the ceiling. Keep leading with your chest as you push your shoulders back and down, away from your ears. Your head should be in line with your spine. Focus forward.

SERIES: 10-second hold

NEED TO MODIFY? Tight hamstrings or back: Sit on the floor with your right leg extended in front of you.

TRANSITION: Slide your right leg back and switch sides; flow into exercise 11.

11. Hip Flexor Stretch (Right)

Repeat exercise 9 with your left leg forward.

TRANSITION: Shift your weight back over your left foot; flow into exercise 12.

12. Hamstring Stretch (Left)

Repeat exercise 10 with your left leg forward.

TRANSITION: Slide your left leg back and kneel down; flow into exercise 13.

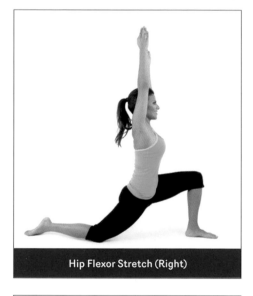

Hip Flexor Stretch (Right)

13. Double Thigh Stretch

FOCUS: Thighs

BREATHING TECHNIQUE: Inhale your hips up and butt forward/Exhale, bend your elbows, and lean back.

GET IN POSITION: Begin by kneeling on the floor and sitting on your heels. Your feet should be comfortably together, with your knees apart and wider than your hips. Place your palms on the floor behind your feet. (Choose a range that is comfortable and turn your hands out for wrist comfort.)

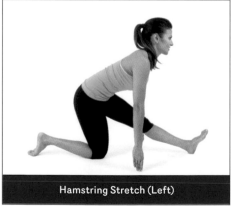

Hamstring Stretch (Left)

Lean back into your hands while lifting your hips and squeezing your butt up. Bend your elbows back as you try to maintain the space between your butt and feet.

SERIES: 5-second hold (Bend your elbows straight back.) 5-second hold, right side (Left arm reaches toward right side.) 5-second hold, left side (Right arm reaches toward left side.) 5-second hold, center (Bend your elbows down as low as you can.)

NEED TO MODIFY? Tender knees: Lie down on your left side. Bend your right knee and take your right hand back, and grab your right foot. Bend your right elbow and pull your foot closer to your butt. Repeat on the other side.

TRANSITION: Lie on your back and slide both of your legs out in front of you; flow into exercise 14.

14. Tucks

FOCUS: Glutes, hips, and inner thighs

INTENTION: "I can have fun right now."

GET IN POSITION: Begin by lying flat on your back. Bend your knees and draw your feet toward your butt, keeping your feet flat on the floor. Keep your feet wider than your hips. (Feel free to play around with your foot placement, closer together or wider apart, to get comfortable.) Turn your knees in slightly. Keep your toes in front of your heels.

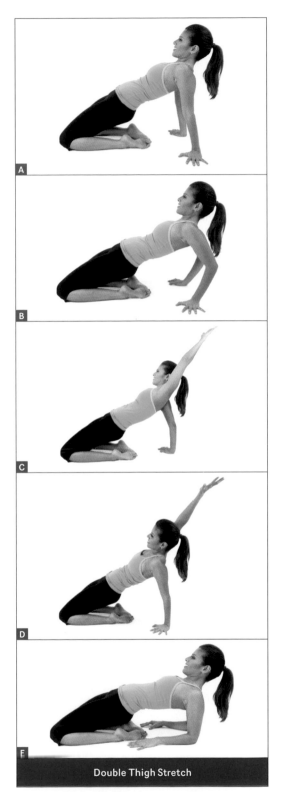

Double Thigh Stretch

GET MOVING: Engage your abs by pulling them in tightly and pushing your back down into the floor. Tucking your pelvis under, press just your butt up and down off the floor. (Try to find a good beat with your butt lifts, like you're bouncing a basketball.) Maintain a small range of motion. (Less is more!) Make sure to keep your abs engaged and your back flat as you isolate just your butt to lift your hips. You're flipping your hips up toward your chest, doing a mini-lift with your butt.

SERIES: 20 single count, *up/down* 20 multi-count, *up/up/up/down* 20 single count, *up/down* 5-second hold

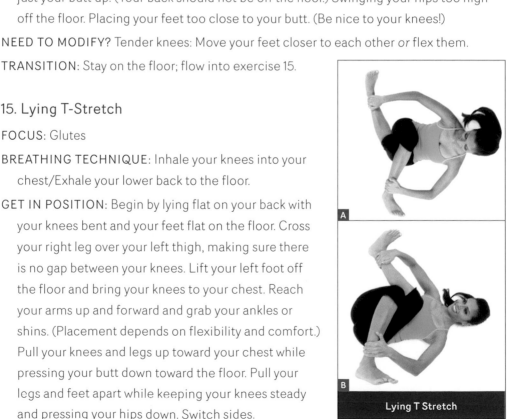

Tucks

LOOK OUT FOR: Using your whole back to lift just your butt up. (Your back should not be off the floor.) Swinging your hips too high off the floor. Placing your feet too close to your butt. (Be nice to your knees!)

NEED TO MODIFY? Tender knees: Move your feet closer to each other *or* flex them.

TRANSITION: Stay on the floor; flow into exercise 15.

15. Lying T-Stretch

FOCUS: Glutes

BREATHING TECHNIQUE: Inhale your knees into your chest/Exhale your lower back to the floor.

GET IN POSITION: Begin by lying flat on your back with your knees bent and your feet flat on the floor. Cross your right leg over your left thigh, making sure there is no gap between your knees. Lift your left foot off the floor and bring your knees to your chest. Reach your arms up and forward and grab your ankles or shins. (Placement depends on flexibility and comfort.) Pull your knees and legs up toward your chest while pressing your butt down toward the floor. Pull your legs and feet apart while keeping your knees steady and pressing your hips down. Switch sides.

Lying T Stretch

SERIES: 10-second hold, right side (right leg on top of left) 10-second hold, left side (left leg on top of right)

NEED TO MODIFY? Tight hips or back: Do Lying 4 Stretch (p. 185).

TRANSITION: Roll over onto your hands and knees; flow into exercise 16.

16. All Fours (Right)

FOCUS: Glutes, hamstrings, and inner thighs

INTENTION: "Less is more; concentrate."

GET IN POSITION: Begin on all fours (on hands and knees) with your feet and knees hip-width apart. Your hands should be a little wider than your shoulders, as if you're setting up for a push-up. Keep your arms straight, pushing away the floor. Tighten your abs by pulling your belly button in toward your spine. Raise your right leg up, getting your knee in line with your hip. Flex your right foot and draw it toward your butt, creating a 90-degree angle with your knee and engaging your hamstring. Keep your back flat and hips level. Shift your weight to the right by leaning into your right palm. While shifting, try to align your left hip with your left knee. Keep your chest open, with your shoulders back and down, away from your ears. Your head should be in line with your spine. Focus on a spot a few inches in front of you on the floor.

GET MOVING: Keep your back flat and stable while lifting your leg up and down. Keep your upper body strong while pushing away the floor. Try to keep your right knee at the same level as your right hip. Engage your hamstring by bending your knee and drawing your right heel toward your butt. To test proper balance, lift your left arm up at any time and make sure your left knee is in line with your left hip. (Keep your left hand in line with your left shoulder, with

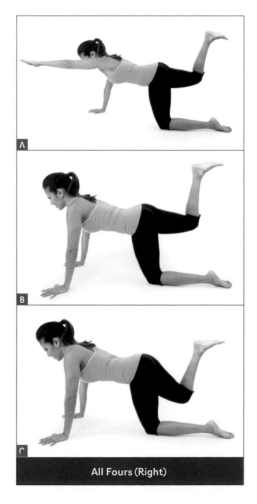

All Fours (Right)

your palm facing down.) Master shifting your weight into your right hand while keeping your hips level.

SERIES: 10-second hold/balance (Lift left arm up.) 20 double count *down/down/up/up* full range (Lower your knee almost to the floor and then lift it to the height of your hip.) 20 single count, *down/up* full range (Lower your knee almost to the floor and then lift it to the level of your hip.) 20 pulses, *up/up* (your knee should remain at hip level.) 10 multi-count, *up/up/up/down* (3 pulses at hip level, then do a single count by moving the knee down to the floor and up to hip level again.) 10 single count, *down/up* full range (knee almost to the floor and then up to hip level.) 10 pulses, *up/up* (your knee should remain at hip level.) 5-second hold/balance (Lift left arm up.)

LOOK OUT FOR: Arching your back. Sinking your weight into your left leg as opposed to shifting it into your right hand. Forgetting to square off your hips. Collapsing your head and shoulders (loose upper body). Swinging your leg, as opposed to making a controlled movement. Lowering your leg too far, or not bringing your leg high enough.

NEED TO MODIFY? Tender wrists or tight shoulders or back: Come to your forearms instead of maintaining straight arms.

TRANSITION: Slide your right leg forward; flow into exercise 17.

17. Pigeon (Right)

FOCUS: Hips and glutes

BREATHING TECHNIQUE: Inhale your left hip down/Exhale your right hip back.

GET IN POSITION: Begin on all fours (on hands and knees) and slide your right knee forward. Make sure your shin is facing out, not tipping down toward the floor. Your right knee should be in line with your right hip. Try to scoot your right foot forward in line with your right knee while anchoring your hips. The more flexible you are, the farther your right foot will be from your groin. Keep your right foot flexed. Keep your back left leg straight, with your toes down and in line with your left hip. Square off your hips, turning your left hip down. Fold your upper body forward, reaching and

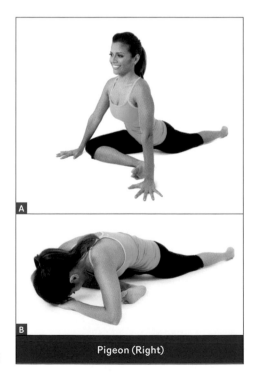

Pigeon (Right)

placing your arms comfortably in front of you. Optional: bring your forehead to the floor.

SERIES: 10-second hold

NEED TO MODIFY? Tender knees: Do Lying T-Stretch or Lying 4 Stretch (p. 185) instead.

TRANSITION: Slide your right leg back; flow into exercise 18.

18. All Fours (Left)

Repeat exercise 16, lifting your left leg.

TRANSITION: Slide your left leg forward; flow into exercise 19.

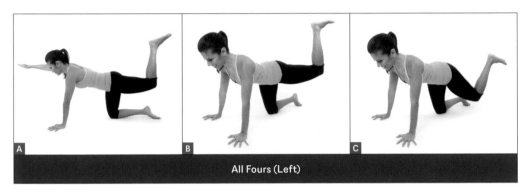

All Fours (Left)

19. Pigeon (Left)

Repeat exercise 17 with your left leg forward.

TRANSITION: Slide your left leg back; flow into exercise 20.

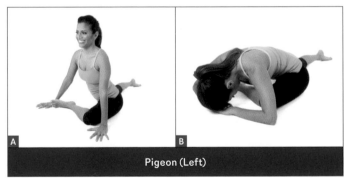

Pigeon (Left)

20. Plank

FOCUS: Core and shoulders

INTENTION: "I can do this. Stay calm and focus on the form."

GET IN POSITION: Begin on all fours (on hands and knees), with your feet and knees hip-width apart. Your hands should be in line with your shoulders, with your palms flat and fingertips spread. Curl your toes under to lift and straighten your legs. Tip your heels forward, as if you are stretching your feet and your body is about to take off. Level your hips and keep your back flat. Tighten your abs by pulling your belly button in toward your spine. Tuck your hips slightly so your back feels protected. Keep your chest open, with your shoulders back and down, away from your ears. Your head should be in line with your spine. Focus on the floor. Your entire body should feel solid, as if you're stuck in a tube.

GET MOVING: Continue to monitor the flatness of your body. Push away from the floor while maintaining good posture. Maintain straight legs. Keep your chest open and your head in line with your spine. Keep shifting your weight forward slightly.

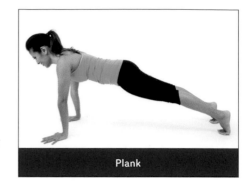

Plank

SERIES: 1-minute hold

LOOK OUT FOR: Keeping your hips too low or too high and arching or rounding your back as a result. Dropping your head. Rounding your shoulders. Placing your hands too close together or too far apart. Placing your hands too far forward and not in line with your shoulders. Arching your back instead of engaging your abs and tucking your hips slightly. Forgetting to tip your heels forward.

NEED TO MODIFY? Tender wrists or tight shoulders: Do Forearm Plank (p. 66) instead. Tender back: Give yourself mini-breaks and be patient.

TRANSITION: Shift your weight and hips back and up; flow into exercise 21.

21. Down Dog

FOCUS: Hamstrings and back

BREATHING TECHNIQUE: Inhale your arms long and hips up/Exhale your shoulders down and heels toward the floor.

GET IN POSITION: Begin in Plank position, make sure your hands are slightly in front of your shoulders. Your palms (parallel or slightly turned out) should be flat and your fingers spread. Keep your toes curled as you shift your weight back and lift your hips up toward the ceiling. As you start to lengthen your arms and legs, continue to press your palms and heels down. As your hips rise toward the ceiling, push the tops of your thighs back and stretch your heels down to the floor, lengthening your hamstrings. Straighten your knees but do not lock them. Maintain straight legs. (Soften your knees if your lower back or hamstrings are tight.) Rotate your elbows in to firm up the arms and shoulders. Maintain

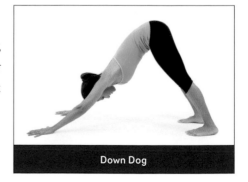

Down Dog

a long back. Keep your head in line with your arms; do not hang your head down. (Note: Imagine you're creating a teepee with your body!)

SERIES: 10-second hold

NEED TO MODIFY? Tender knees or tight back and hamstrings: Keep your legs bent and heels raised.

TRANSITION: Lower your hips and shift your weight forward and hands wider; flow into exercise 22.

22. Push-Ups

FOCUS: Chest, arms, and core

INTENTION: "Even if it is tiny, it counts—and I'm getting stronger."

GET IN POSITION: Begin in Plank position with your hands wider than your shoulders, palms flat and fingertips spread. Keep your feet hip-width apart. Straighten your legs. Tip your heels forward, as if you are stretching your feet and your body is about to take off. Level your hips and keep your back flat. Tighten your abs by pulling your belly button in toward your spine. Tuck your hips slightly so your back feels protected. Keep your chest open, with your shoulders back and down, away from your ears. Your head should be in line with your spine. Focus on the floor. Your entire body should feel solid, as if you're stuck in a tube.

GET MOVING: Bending your elbows and leading with your chest, lower your entire body down to the floor and then straighten your arms to lift your entire body back up. Lower yourself as far to the floor as you can without sacrificing your form—even a mini push-up counts! Make sure you keep tipping your heels forward with every push-up. Maintain good posture and tap into your core strength for this workout.

SERIES: 20 single count, *down/up*

LOOK OUT FOR: Keeping your hips too low or too high and arching or rounding your back as a result. Dropping your head. Rounding your shoulders and not squeezing your shoulder blades together on the way down. Placing your hands too close together or too far apart. Placing your hands too far forward and not in line with

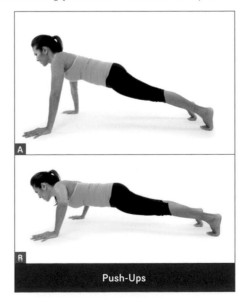

Push-Ups

your shoulders. Arching your back instead of engaging your abs and tucking your hips slightly. Forgetting to tip your heels forward. Giving up because you can manage only a tiny range of movement.

NEED TO MODIFY? Tender wrists or tight shoulders: Make fists and substitute them for your flat palms. Tender back: Give yourself mini-breaks and be patient *or* do Push-Up Bent Knees (p. 88) instead.

TRANSITION: Shift your weight and hips back and up; flow into exercise 23.

23. Down Dog

Repeat exercise 21.

TRANSITION: Shift your weight forward; flow into exercise 24.

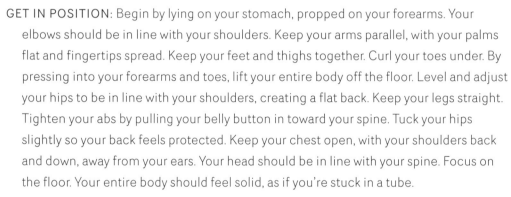

Down Dog

24. Forearm Plank

FOCUS: Core and shoulders

INTENTION: "I'm here; if I think I'm strong, so will my body."

GET IN POSITION: Begin by lying on your stomach, propped on your forearms. Your elbows should be in line with your shoulders. Keep your arms parallel, with your palms flat and fingertips spread. Keep your feet and thighs together. Curl your toes under. By pressing into your forearms and toes, lift your entire body off the floor. Level and adjust your hips to be in line with your shoulders, creating a flat back. Keep your legs straight. Tighten your abs by pulling your belly button in toward your spine. Tuck your hips slightly so your back feels protected. Keep your chest open, with your shoulders back and down, away from your ears. Your head should be in line with your spine. Focus on the floor. Your entire body should feel solid, as if you're stuck in a tube.

GET MOVING: Continue to monitor the flatness of your body. Push away from the floor while maintaining good posture. Keep your legs straight. Keep your chest open and your head in line with your spine. Continue to shift your weight forward slightly.

SERIES: 1-minute hold

LOOK OUT FOR: Keeping your hips too low or too high and arching or rounding your back as a result. Dropping your head. Rounding your shoulders. Sticking your butt up instead of engaging your abs and keeping a flat

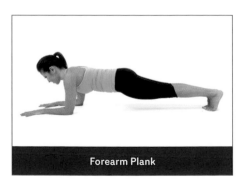

Forearm Plank

back. Arching your back instead of engaging your abs and tucking your hips slightly. Forgetting to maintain strong legs.

NEED TO MODIFY? Tender back: Give yourself mini-breaks and be patient *or* do Plank (p. 63) instead.

TRANSITION: Lower your knees, shift your weight, and rest back; flow into exercise 25.

25. Child's Pose with Arm Extension

FOCUS: Shoulders and chest

BREATHING TECHNIQUE: Inhale your arms up and forward toward your head/Exhale your lower back and hips down.

GET IN POSITION: Begin by kneeling on the floor and sitting on your heels. Your feet should be comfortably together, with your knees apart and wider than your hips. Fold your upper body forward between your thighs and bring your forehead to the floor. Clasp your hands together behind your back and reach your arms straight up toward the ceiling and forward toward your head. Rock your arms from side to side.

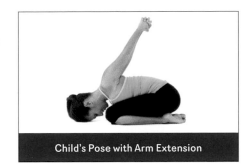

Child's Pose with Arm Extension

SERIES: 10-second hold

NEED TO MODIFY? Tender knees: Place a pillow under your hamstrings for elevation or play around with the placement of your knees until you feel comfortable.

TRANSITION: Roll your body up and bring your legs out in front of you; flow into exercise 26.

26. Clam/Forearm Plank Interval

FOCUS: Core

INTENTION: "I'm going to attack this interval."

GET IN POSITION: Begin by sitting on the floor with your hands placed comfortably behind your back. Your hands should be placed wider than your shoulders, palms flat and fingertips turned out. Bend your knees and draw your feet toward your butt, keeping your feet flat on the floor. Keep your feet and knees together. (Feel free to play around with your knee placement, holding them closer together or wider apart to get comfortable.) Keep your toes in front of your heels. Lean into your hands and bend your elbows slightly to lift your legs off the floor. Balance on your butt and hands with your bent legs in the air. Flex your feet. Make sure your back muscles feel solid and your abs are engaged and anchored in. Keep your shoulders back and down. Lean back, bend your elbows more, and push your knees away (straighten your legs if you can) and then bend your knees in toward your chest as you straighten your arms and lean your upper body forward. Repeat this *out* and *in* motion—the "clam." Just after completing the clam part of the series, flip over immediately into a Forearm Plank.

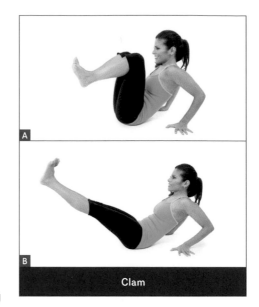

GET MOVING: *Clam:* Make sure to open your body by leaning back and then close your body by leaning forward. Maintain your balance on your butt; be aware of engaging your abs and not your back to open and close your legs. (Your range of movement will depend on your comfort and strength.) *Forearm Plank:* Make sure to maintain your form (flat back!) even though the transitions are fast. To ensure a challenge, maintain quick transitions as you alternate between Clam and Forearm Plank.

Clam

SERIES: **Set 1:** *Clam:* 20 single count, *open/close Forearm Plank:* 5-second hold 20 single count pikes *up/down* (make a teepee with your body, shifting your weight out of your shoulders up to ceiling, as in Down Dog) 10-second hold **Set 2:** *Clam:* 20 single count, *open/close Forearm Plank:* 5-second hold 20 single count, *bend/stretch* (bend and stretch the knees to straight legs/make sure bends are tiny) 10-second hold

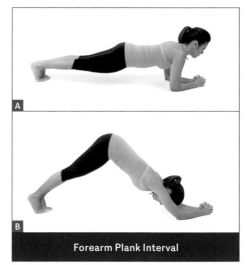

Forearm Plank Interval

LOOK OUT FOR: *Clam:* Getting the choreography mixed up. (Make sure to fully open and close the legs in conjunction with your upper body leaning back and forward.) Collapsing your chest. Using your hips to move instead of engaging your abs. Forgetting to concentrate on your abs generating the workout. *Forearm Plank:* Keeping your hips too low or too high and arching or rounding your back as a result. Dropping your head. Rounding your shoulders. Sticking your butt up instead of engaging your abs and keeping a flat back. Arching your back instead of engaging your abs and tucking your hips slightly. Forgetting to maintain strong legs.

NEED TO MODIFY? Tender back (Clam): Rest on your forearms and raise your legs up instead of balancing on your butt; continue the out-and-in motion with your legs only. Tender back (Forearm Plank): Give yourself mini-breaks and be patient *or* do Plank (p. 63) instead.

TRANSITION: Slowly lower your body; flow into exercise 27.

27. Cobra

FOCUS: Core and back

BREATHING TECHNIQUE: Inhale your chest up/Exhale your hips forward and shoulders back.

GET IN POSITION: Begin by lying on your stomach, propped on your forearms. Slide your hands back under your shoulders, keeping your palms flat and fingertips spread. Keep your elbows bent, hugging them tightly into your body. Keep your feet and knees hip-width apart. Press the tops of your feet, thighs, and hips firmly into the floor. Start to lengthen and straighten your arms while lifting your chest off the floor. Keep your shoulder blades back, puffing your ribs forward. Keep your hips connected to the floor and lift your upper body. (You might not be able to straighten your arms entirely, so feel free to keep your elbows slightly bent for comfort.) Firm up your butt and drive your hips forward while lifting your chest and stretching your abs. Twist your upper body to the right and to the left, lengthening your sides, and then return to center. (Repeat the movement twice.)

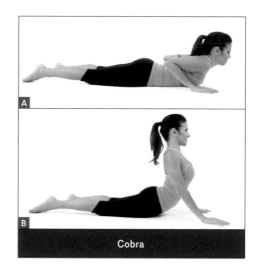
Cobra

SERIES: 10-second hold

NEED TO MODIFY? Tender back: Do Cat/Cow (p. 99) instead.

TRANSITION: Lower; flow into exercise 28.

28. Superman

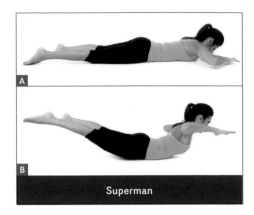

Superman

FOCUS: Back

INTENTION: "I'm creating a stronger back. My posture will improve."

GET IN POSITION: Begin by lying on your stomach, resting your forehead on your hands. Keep your feet and knees hip-width apart. Engage and straighten your legs as you point your toes. Stretch your arms forward a little wider than your shoulders. Keep a slight bend in your elbows. Your palms should be facing down. Tighten your abs by pulling your belly button in toward your spine Your head should be slightly above the floor. Try to keep your head in line with your spine. (Don't crank your head up!) Focus on the floor.

GET MOVING: Lift and lower your arms and legs using your back/posture muscles. Squeeze your shoulder blades together and your butt slightly as your chest and legs rise on the way up. Keep your abs and back engaged as you lower your arms and legs.

SERIES: 20 single count, *up/down* 5-second hold

LOOK OUT FOR: Lifting your head instead of your arms and stressing your neck muscles. Not lifting your chest and legs high enough on the rise. Placing your feet too far apart. Forgetting to target your back muscles.

NEED TO MODIFY? Tender back: Lift up and down in Cobra (p. 69) instead.

TRANSITION: Shift your weight and rest back; flow into exercise 29.

29. Child's Pose

FOCUS: Shoulders and back

MANTRA: The solution is born before the problem.

BREATHING TECHNIQUE: Inhale and exhale; observe your chest rising and falling. Embrace a sense of calm.

GET IN POSITION: Begin by kneeling on the floor and sitting on your heels. Your feet should be comfortably together, with your knees apart and wider than your hips. Fold your upper body forward between your

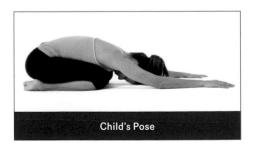

Child's Pose

thighs and bring your forehead to the floor. Reach your straight arms forward with your palms down. Release your shoulders toward the floor.

SERIES: 10-second hold

NEED TO MODIFY? Tender knees: Place a pillow under your hamstrings for elevation *or* play around with the placement of your knees until you feel comfortable.

TRANSITION: Roll your body up and open your legs in front of you; flow into exercise 30.

30. Seated Straddle

FOCUS: Inner thighs and back

MANTRA: The solution is born before the problem.

BREATHING TECHNIQUE: Inhale and reach your arms forward/Exhale and ground your hips down and back. Embrace your new drive.

GET IN POSITION: Sit on your floor with your legs straight and spread as far apart as your flexibility allows. Use your hands to push your hips forward and keep your legs in a wide V-shape. Keep your knees parallel and facing up toward the ceiling; point your toes. Lift your left arm up toward the ceiling and reach over to the right. Lean your upper body to the right as you twist your chest open toward the ceiling. Repeat on the other side with your right arm reaching. After both sides, return to center and reach your arms straight out in front of you. Walk your fingertips forward as you fold your upper body down toward the floor, hinging at your hips.

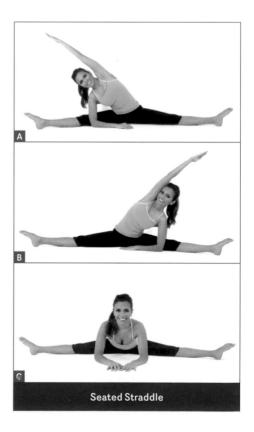

Seated Straddle

SERIES: 10-second hold, right side (Left arm reaches toward right side.) 10-second hold, left side (Right arm reaches toward left side.) 10-second hold, center (Reach both arms straight forward through the center.)

NEED TO MODIFY? Tight groin or hips: Fold your mat a little and use it as a cushion under your butt and/or create a smaller V-shape with your legs.

THE POST-WORKOUT

1 **Post-Workout Recap:**

Be proud of yourself. You took your anger and channeled its powerful energy toward a productive, solution-focused workout.

Did my emotional weight change?

☐ YES ☐ NO

Did I accomplish my workout intention?

☐ YES ☐ NO

Is there a change in my physical body?

☐ YES ☐ NO

2 **My Post-Workout Mood Is:**

(Write down, think, or say out loud.)

_____

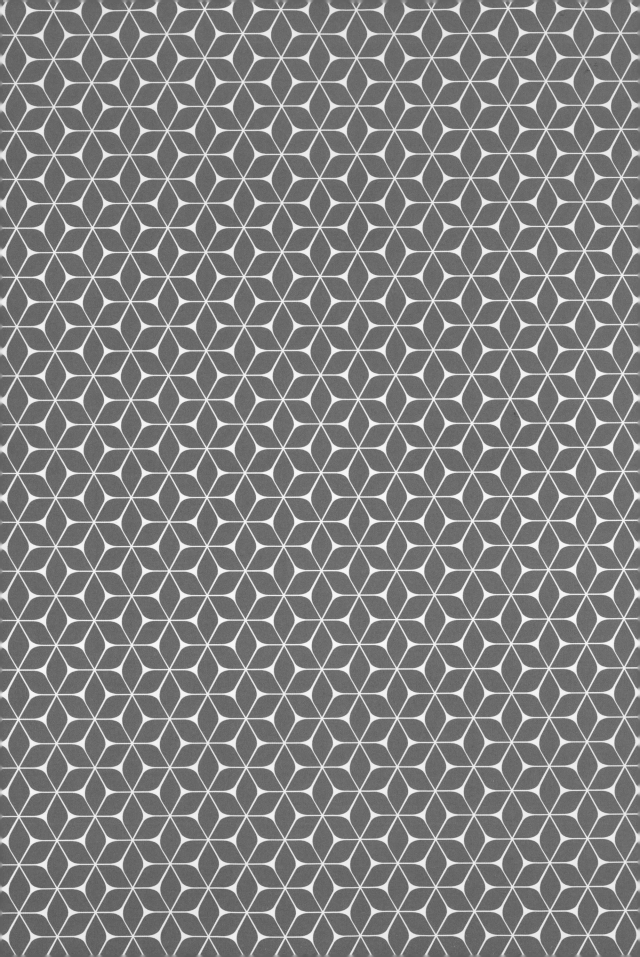

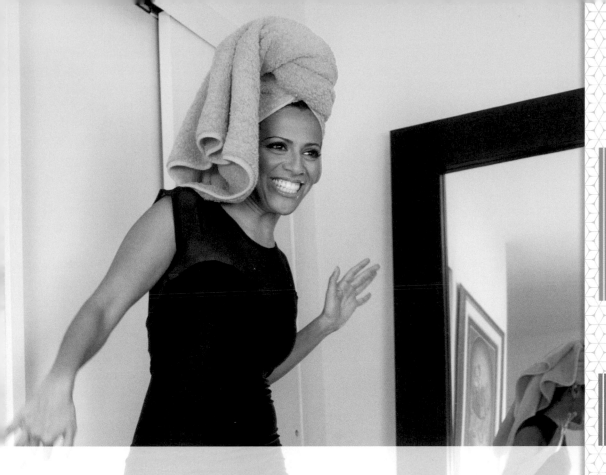

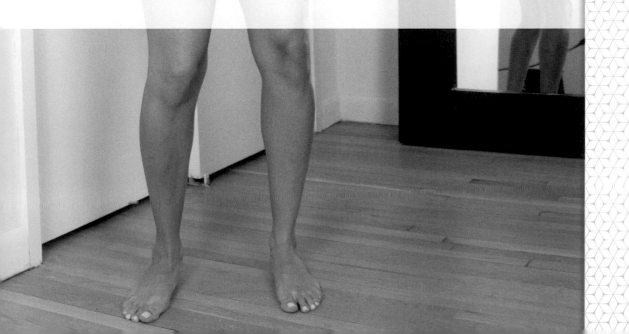

— CHAPTER 4 —

THE ENERGY WORKOUT

THE ENERGY EXERCISES

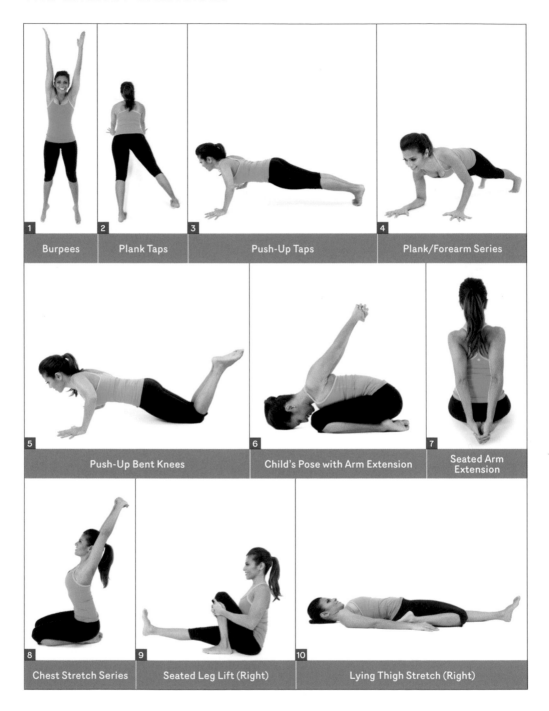

1. Burpees
2. Plank Taps
3. Push-Up Taps
4. Plank/Forearm Series
5. Push-Up Bent Knees
6. Child's Pose with Arm Extension
7. Seated Arm Extension
8. Chest Stretch Series
9. Seated Leg Lift (Right)
10. Lying Thigh Stretch (Right)

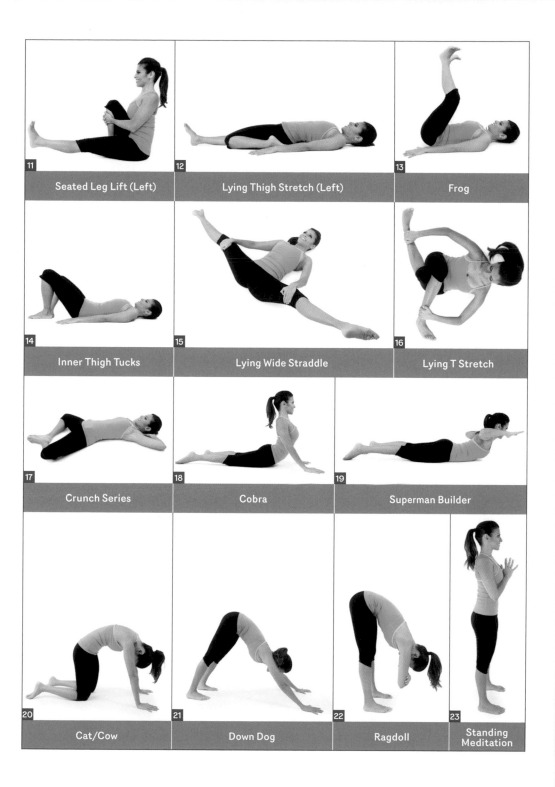

11 — Seated Leg Lift (Left)

12 — Lying Thigh Stretch (Left)

13 — Frog

14 — Inner Thigh Tucks

15 — Lying Wide Straddle

16 — Lying T Stretch

17 — Crunch Series

18 — Cobra

19 — Superman Builder

20 — Cat/Cow

21 — Down Dog

22 — Ragdoll

23 — Standing Meditation

Energy is fuel. It can ignite action, move you toward a goal, and unlock your potential. You feel invincible. Fuel plus drive is a superpotent combination.

That being said, energy has a flip side. Too much energy can leave you scatterbrained, exhausted, and even manic. A crash could be looming on the horizon, especially when your energy isn't balanced or properly channeled. Think about where you are on the energy spectrum and why.

What is the emotional weight of your energy and its resulting mood, and how is it manifesting in your physical body?

THE PRE-WORKOUT

1 **I Am Feeling:**

☐ Able	☐ Euphoric	☐ Potent
☐ Buoyant	☐ Excited	☐ Powerful
☐ Capable	☐ Exhilarated	☐ Productive
☐ Certain	☐ Exuberant	☐ Quick
☐ Challenged	☐ Firm	☐ Risky
☐ Competent	☐ Forceful	☐ Secure
☐ Confident	☐ Frisky	☐ Sound
☐ Determined	☐ Full of gusto	☐ Spirited
☐ Dynamic	☐ Impatient	☐ Stable
☐ Ebullient	☐ Impregnable	☐ Steadfast
☐ Effective	☐ Indomitable	☐ Strong
☐ Effervescent	☐ Invigorated	☐ Sturdy
☐ Efficient	☐ Invincible	☐ Successful
☐ Empowered	☐ Jaunty	☐ Unbeatable
☐ Enabled	☐ Manic	☐ Unlimited
☐ Encouraged	☐ Mighty	☐ Vigorous
☐ Energized	☐ Overexerted	☐ Vital
☐ Enthusiastic	☐ Perky	☐ Vivacious

Choose from the list above, or add your own words. Then write down your mood *or* say it out loud and embrace it.

2 My Current Mood Is:

_____

3 My Emotional Weight Is:

1	5	10
Light	Neutral	Heavy

4 My Physical Symptoms Are:

- ☐ Adrenaline Rush
- ☐ Agitation
- ☐ Alertness
- ☐ Bounciness
- ☐ Confident Movement
- ☐ Easy Digestion
- ☐ Endorphin Release
- ☐ Flushing
- ☐ Fidgeting
- ☐ Glowing

- ☐ Goosebumps
- ☐ Head Rubbing
- ☐ Hunger
- ☐ Hyperfocused
- ☐ Increased Breathing
- ☐ Increased Dopamine
- ☐ Insomnia
- ☐ Jerkiness
- ☐ Jitteriness
- ☐ Manic Energy

- ☐ Open Posture
- ☐ Pacing
- ☐ Rapid Heartbeat
- ☐ Shaking
- ☐ Smiling
- ☐ Sparkling
- ☐ Sweating
- ☐ Talkative
- ☐ Tingling
- ☐ Toe-Tapping

TEN COMMON ENERGY THOUGHTS

- I think I'll run another mile today because I feel so good.
- Sure, I can do that task for you. I'm so glad you asked and I can help you out today.
- I'm a yes person today—somehow I feel like I can take on the world. Go ahead and throw it at me!
- Nothing's better than a good, deep sleep to get me ready for a vigorous day.
- I hope I feel like this all the time, because having this kind of confidence is really empowering.
- You want to go hiking this weekend? Why not?
- Okay, I'm done putting it off. Today I am finally going to clean out those closets.
- Jeez, I'm like the Energizer Bunny: I keep going and going!
- Nothing can stop me. I can will my way through anything today.
- Bring it on!

1 **Mantra for Energy:**

Let go. Live. Love.

I love being filled with energy. When it's right, it feels like I've been eating the healthiest food and downing the freshest of juices since birth. I feel *unstoppable*.

I know it's impossible but I want to feel that way all the time, as energy is one of my favorite moods. When I'm energized, I want to bottle up my electricity and share it over and over again. In that moment, capturing the forces and stars that must have aligned to create my incredible high actually seems doable. And I've learned that this mantra, "Let go. Live. Love," is the biggest resource we have to get closer to feeling this way all the time.

Being energized is like being in a perfect storm in the very best possible way. You want to embrace living and loving. This is what makes this mood the ideal time to not only feel powerful but also tackle any loose ends in your life that typically weigh you down. The things and people we hold on to usually take away our energy, and more often than not, our increased energy has come from letting go of something or someone. The "Let go. Live. Love" mantra reaffirms the power of letting go even when letting go seems impossible, and explores the energy-zapping consequences of holding on.

Take what happened with my beloved older brother, my only sibling. After several years in corporate America, this analytical, practical, smart, and experienced young man decided to go work for my father in his heating and air-conditioning business. This was my dad's dream: his only son, whom he respected and loved greatly, choosing the family business over a corporate job! Filled with big ideas and much excitement about this father/son venture, my father couldn't have been happier.

It started out well, but like many other family businesses, the working relationship was complicated and quickly became negative as repressed emotions came out. My mom felt that the stresses between father and son could become dangerous to their close relationship. So, in what she believed was the best interest of the family, she fired my brother, but not without offering to support him financially for as long as he needed. My brother, shocked and enraged, was so devastated he refused to talk to my parents for three long years. Three years!

This family experience still astonishes me. I was still living with my parents during most of this time and never once heard or felt a sense of regret, anger, judgment, or lack of faith that my brother would eventually speak to them again. How did they let go of such a painful situation, seemingly just like that? Didn't they feel as if he was overreacting? How did they go from seeing and talking to my brother every single day to not at all? Didn't they feel like proving a point or guilt-tripping my brother for his behavior? They *didn't*.

My mom had faith in herself and my brother. She honored the noncommunication and created room in her heart so she could truly listen to my brother when he was ready to speak to her again. Armed with the energy to be patient, she was able to genuinely let go of her desire to control the situation.

For her, truly letting go means accepting people, situations, and realities rather than holding on to them. Sometimes we falsely let go, thinking we've moved on when, in actuality, we're still trying to maintain control. My mom might have learned to put up with my brother's distance, but the heaviness of the situation would have been rehashed over and over again to no good purpose. By just *dealing* with it and merely getting used to the distance, she wouldn't have truly accepted his choice and it could have been detrimental to their relationship in the future. And conversely, had my brother been evasive and continued in a stressed relationship, it might have led to their bond being severed forever. He had to take time to let go of the failed partnership, to eventually recycle that energy toward the rebirth of an even better relationship with my parents.

Think about the alternatives to the actions of this mantra. They are hold on, die, and hate.

Holding on, as opposed to letting go, causes a lack of movement and intense feelings (often of negativity or hate) and manifests in a life lacking vigor and vitality (a death of energy). It is guaranteed to zap your energy and, at its worst, zap your life. If you want to live a happy life, you must let go of the tight grip you can easily have on the numerous things in life that could deplete your energy: a friend not calling back, a mean comment, a stranger stealing your parking space, a job lost, a date flaking, loved ones not understanding you.

Life happens. You'll make mistakes; others will make mistakes. You'll ask for forgiveness; others will ask you for forgiveness. You'll want to be loved; others will want you to love them. You'll want people to listen; others will want you to listen. Stuff happens and more stuff will happen. Holding on depletes you of the energy needed to be as happy as you could possibly be.

Learning this enlightened lesson can be the best possible use of your energy. This mantra has led to my parents and brother having one of the most special and honest relationships I've ever seen.

As my mom would say, life has a cycle. "Let go. Live. Love" is a cyclical lesson.

To *let go*, you must *live* and *love*.

To *live*, you must *let go* and *love*.

To *love*, you must *let go* and *live*.

And the cycle will continue.

Even though I've been hurt, made mistakes, felt misunderstood, and have the ability to defend and fight back, I can choose a different route. And, especially when I'm energized, I choose to let go. I choose to live and love. I choose to fill my life with added boosts of movement and the knowledge that life is an ever-evolving, unpredictable process, and when I have energy I want to savor, spread, and capitalize on every bit of it.

2 How to Use the Mantra

The overall theme here is to use your energy wisely. Try not to empty the tank or save all your fuel for a rainy day: ration it out. Find the ideal use for your energy's power by striking a balance between letting go and holding on.

That is what this mantra can help you do. You want to harness your energy for sustainability and fulfillment. Use your energy to free yourself of holding on—let go of old, self-critical patterns or painful experiences—and channel that immense burst of productivity toward long-term benefits. "Let go. Live. Love" is about becoming an open bubble, buoyant and balanced, waiting to be filled up with love and happiness, without any emotional weight pulling you back down to earth. Your spirit wants to be vibrant, hopeful, and have room to receive good things. When that happens, it's almost as if your mind and body are working in perfect tandem, telling you that all is well in the world.

Repeat the "Let go. Live. Love" mantra, enjoy your newfound energy, and let your body go so you can relish a vibrant and active workout.

3 Why the Energy Workout

By now you have taken the time to reflect on the source and scope of your energy and how it is weighing on you emotionally and physically.

The flow of this series is designed for you to tap into that energy to do a lot of reps and stay in constant motion. Move, move, move!

Embrace your mood, reflect on the mantra, and let it provide you with even more energy to liven up this vibrant and super-fueled routine.

4 **My Energy Workout Intention (Emotional or Physical) Is:**

(Write down, think, or say out loud.)

_____

MUSIC

Choose music that will capitalize on your energy and help add fun fuel to your fire. Here are a few suggestions that will keep that blood flowing:

1960s: "Respect" ▪ Aretha Franklin

1970s: "Superstition" ▪ Stevie Wonder

1980s: "Eye of the Tiger" ▪ Survivor

1990s: "We Like to Party" ▪ Venga Boys

2000s: "Fire Burning" ▪ Sean Kingston

2010s: "Can't Hold Us" ▪ Macklemore & Ryan Lewis

---

5 **The Energy Exercises**

1. Burpees

FOCUS: Total body cardio

INTENTION: "Let me tap into my energy and let it flow through my body."

GET IN POSITION: Be familiar with the one basic Burpee flow: 1. Begin in Standing Meditation. 2. Bend down and jump back into a Plank. (Place your hands on the floor with your knees bent and then jump.) 3. Immediately jump your feet from Plank back between your hands. 4. Return to stand and swing your arms up toward the ceiling. 5. Jump up and land in Standing Meditation.

GET MOVING: Repeat steps 2–4 and try to maintain speed. When jumping up, reach your arms toward the ceiling. Land in a strong squat with your palms flat on the floor. Immediately jump back into a strong plank with your abs engaged and your back flat. Evenly hop forward and spring back up again.

SERIES: 15 single count (Jumping up once completes one burpee.)

LOOK OUT FOR: Not flattening your palms on the floor for the squat/plank. Favoring one side of your body over the other. Keeping your hips too low or too high and arching or rounding your back as a result. Dropping your head. Rounding your shoulders. Placing your hands too close together or too far apart. Placing your hands too far forward and not in line with your shoulders. Being bouncy in your movements instead of controlled. Arching your back instead of engaging your abs and tucking your hips slightly. Forgetting to tip your heels forward.

NEED TO MODIFY? Tender knees or back: Skip the jumping and step back into Plank one leg at a time.

TRANSITION: On the last burpee, jump into and stay in Plank; flow into exercise 2.

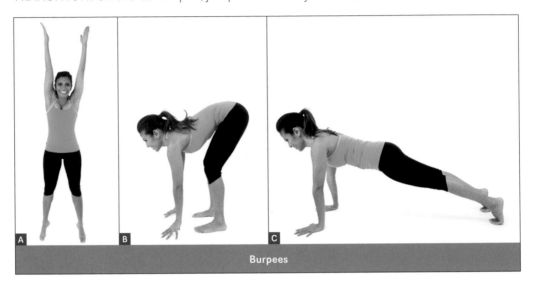

Burpees

2. Plank Taps

FOCUS: Core and shoulders

INTENTION: "I can do this. Stay calm and focus on the form."

GET IN POSITION: Begin in Plank with your hands in line with your shoulders, palms flat and fingertips spread. Keep your feet and thighs together. Straighten your legs. Tip your heels forward, as if you are stretching your feet and your body is about to take off. Level your hips and keep your back flat. Tighten your abs by pulling your belly button in toward your spine. Tuck your hips slightly so your back feels protected. Keep your chest open, with your shoulders back and down, away from your ears. Your head should be in line with your spine. Focus on the floor. Your entire body should feel solid, as if you're stuck in a tube.

GET MOVING: Continue to monitor the flatness of your body. Push away from the floor while maintaining good posture. Maintain straight legs. Keeping your right leg straight, tap your right foot out to the right side and then bring it back to center. Repeat the movement on your left side. Make sure to keep the leg that is not moving straight.

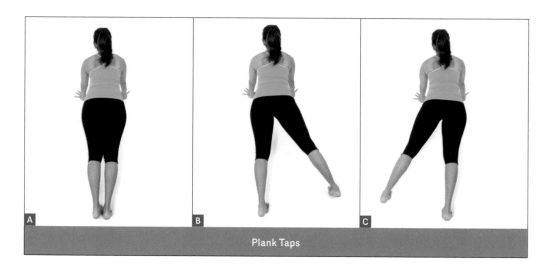

Plank Taps

Keep your chest open and your head in line with your spine. Keep shifting your weight forward slightly.

SERIES: 5-second hold 10 single count taps *right/center/left/center* (Tempo is key!) 10-second hold

LOOK OUT FOR: Keeping your hips too low or too high and arching or rounding your back as a result. Dropping your head. Rounding your shoulders. Placing your hands too close together or too far apart. Placing your hands too far forward and not in line with your shoulders. Bending your legs when tapping instead of keeping your legs straight. Arching your back instead of engaging your abs and tucking your hips slightly. Forgetting to tip your heels forward.

NEED TO MODIFY? Tender wrists or shoulders: Do Forearm Plank (p. 66) instead. Tender back: Give yourself mini-breaks and be patient *or* skip the taps and just hold.

TRANSITION: Take a quick breather; flow into exercise 3.

3. Push-Up Taps

FOCUS: Chest, arms, and core

INTENTION: "Even if it is tiny, it counts—and I'm getting stronger."

GET IN POSITION: Begin in Plank with your hands wider than your shoulders, palms flat and fingertips spread. Keep your feet and thighs together. Straighten your legs. Tip your heels forward, as if you are stretching your feet and your body is about to take off. Level your hips and keep your back flat. Tighten your abs by pulling your belly button in toward your spine. Tuck your hips slightly so your back feels protected. Keep your chest open, with your shoulders back and down, away from your ears. Your head should be in line with your spine. Focus on the floor. Your entire body should feel solid, as if you're stuck in a tube.

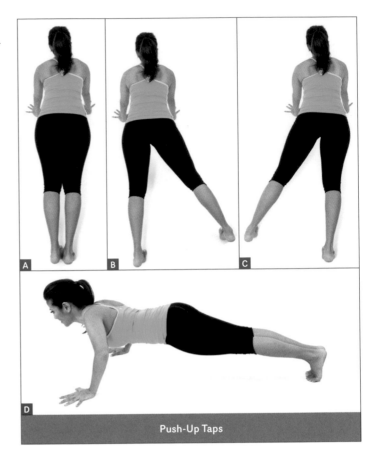

Push-Up Taps

GET MOVING: Keeping your right leg straight, tap your right foot out to the right side and then bring it back to center. Repeat the movement on your left side. After the right and left taps, do a push-up by bending your elbows, lowering your entire body down to the floor, and then straightening your arms to lift your entire body back up. Leading with your chest, lower yourself as far as you can without sacrificing your form—even a mini push-up counts! Make sure you keep tipping your heels forward with every push-up. Maintain good posture and tap into your core strength for this workout.

SERIES: 10 single count tap push-ups (right and left taps followed by a push-up) 10 single count push-ups *down/up*

LOOK OUT FOR: Keeping your hips too low or too high and arching or rounding your back as a result. Dropping your head. Rounding your shoulders. Placing your hands too close together or too far apart. Placing your hands too far forward and not in line with your shoulders. Bending your legs when tapping instead of keeping your legs straight. Moving too fast. Arching your back instead of engaging your abs and tucking your hips slightly. Forgetting to tip your heels forward.

NEED TO MODIFY? Tender wrists or tight shoulders: Make fists and substitute them for your flat palms. Tender back: Give yourself mini-breaks and be patient *or* do Push-Up Bent Knees (p. 88) instead.

TRANSITION: Take a quick breather; flow into exercise 4.

4. Plank/Forearm Series

FOCUS: Core and shoulders

INTENTION: "Let me zero in on my potential and do this!"

GET IN POSITION: Series moves back and forth between Plank (straight-arm) and Forearm Plank. Begin in Plank position with your hands in line with your shoulders, palms flat and fingertips spread. Keep your feet hip-width apart. Straighten your legs. Tip your heels forward, as if you are stretching your feet and your body is about to take off. Level your hips and keep your back flat. Tighten your abs by pulling your belly button in toward your spine. Tuck your hips slightly so your back feels protected. Keep your chest open, with your shoulders back and down, away from your ears. Your head should be in line with your spine. Focus on the floor. Your entire body should feel solid, as if you're stuck in a tube.

GET MOVING: Continue to monitor the flatness of your body. Push away from the floor while maintaining good posture. Maintain straight legs. Lower your right forearm onto the floor and then your left forearm (into a Forearm Plank). Then, press your right hand down into the floor and straight your right arm as you press your left hand down into the floor to straighten your left arm, returning into a Plank. Repeat the movement, starting with your left forearm. Keep your chest open and your head in line with your spine. Keep shifting your weight forward slightly. Maintain your attention to detail while moving from Plank to Forearm Plank.

SERIES: 5-second hold 5 single count, *down/down/up/up* (right forearm start) 5 single count, *down/down/up/up* (left forearm start)

LOOK OUT FOR: Keeping your hips too low or too high and arching or rounding your back as a result. Dropping your head. Rounding your shoulders. Placing your hands too close together or too far apart. Placing your hands too far forward and not in line with your shoulders. Swinging your body and using momentum,

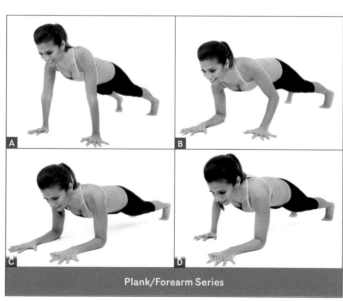

Plank/Forearm Series

instead of control and strength to get through the movements. Arching your back instead of engaging your abs and tucking your hips slightly. Forgetting to tip your heels forward.

NEED TO MODIFY? Tender back: Give yourself mini-breaks and be patient *or* stay in Plank for 1 minute and then in Forearm Plank for 1 minute.

TRANSITION: Take a quick breather while staying on your hands and knees; flow into exercise 5.

5. Push-Up Bent Knees

FOCUS: Chest, arms, and core

GET IN POSITION: Begin on all fours (on hands and knees) with your hands wider than your shoulders, palms flat and fingertips spread. Keep your feet and knees together. Shift your hips forward, lifting your feet up toward your butt, and point your toes. Keep your arms straight. Tighten your abs by pulling your belly button in toward your spine. Tuck your hips slightly so your back feels protected. Keep your chest open, with your shoulders back and down, away from your ears. Your head should be in line with your spine. Focus on the floor. Your entire body should feel solid and strong.

GET MOVING: Bending your elbows and leading with your chest, lower your entire body to the floor and then straighten your arms to lift your entire upper body back up. Lower yourself as far as you can without sacrificing your form—even a mini push-up counts! Make sure you keep pulling your feet up toward your butt. Maintain good posture and tap into your core strength for this workout.

SERIES: 10 double count, *down/down/up/up*
10 single count, *down/up*

LOOK OUT FOR: Keeping your hips too low or too high and arching or rounding your back as a result. Dropping your head. Rounding your shoulders and not squeezing your shoulder blades together on the way down. Placing your hands too close together or too far apart. Placing your hands too far forward and not in line with your shoulders. Arching your back instead of engaging your abs and tucking your hips slightly. Favoring one arm over the other and not pushing into both hands evenly. Forgetting

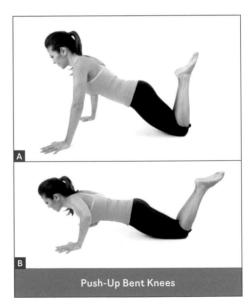

A

B

Push-Up Bent Knees

to pull your feet up. Giving up because you can manage only a tiny range of movement. Rushing your movement and not following the tempo.

NEED TO MODIFY? Tender wrists and tight shoulders: Make fists and substitute them for your flat palms. Tender back: Give yourself mini-breaks and be patient *or* do push-ups against the wall.

TRANSITION: Shift your weight and rest back; flow into exercise 6.

6. Child's Pose with Arm Extension

FOCUS: Shoulders and chest

BREATHING TECHNIQUE: Inhale your arms up and forward toward your head/Exhale your lower back and hips down.

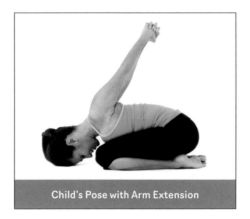

Child's Pose with Arm Extension

GET IN POSITION: Begin by kneeling on the floor and sitting on your heels. Your feet should be comfortably together, with your knees apart and wider than your hips. Fold your upper body forward between your thighs and bring your forehead to the floor. Clasp your hands together behind your back and reach your arms straight up toward the ceiling and forward toward your head. Rock your arms from side to side.

SERIES: 10-second hold

NEED TO MODIFY? Tender knees: Place a pillow under your hamstrings for elevation *or* play around with the placement of your knees until you feel comfortable.

TRANSITION: Roll your upper body up and stay seated on your feet; flow into exercise 7.

7. Seated Arm Extension

FOCUS: Arms, shoulders, and chest

BREATHING TECHNIQUE: Inhale your chest up/Exhale your shoulders down.

GET IN POSITION: Begin by kneeling on the floor and sitting on your heels. (This is basically the same as exercise 6, but you're sitting up.) Your feet should be comfortably together, with your knees apart and wider than your hips. Clasp your hands firmly as you interlace your fingers together behind your back. Reach your knuckles down toward the floor and back behind you. Lean back as you lengthen your abs and chest up and away from your hips. Continue to reach your arms back as you lift your chest up higher.

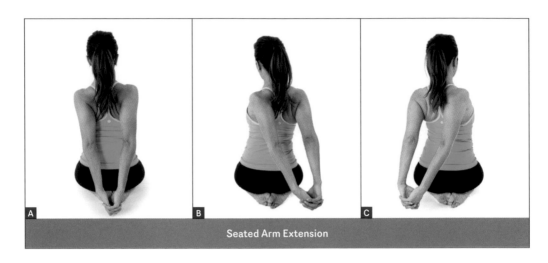

Seated Arm Extension

Maintain good posture and keep leaning back. (Avoid the temptation to lean forward.) Your head should be in line with your spine. Focus forward. Rock your arms side to side.

SERIES: 10-second hold

NEED TO MODIFY? Tender knees: Place a pillow under your hamstrings for elevation *or* play around with placement of your knees.

TRANSITION: Unhook your hands and stay seated; flow into exercise 8.

8. Chest Stretch Series

FOCUS: Arms, shoulders, and chest

BREATHING TECHNIQUE: Inhale your arms up/Exhale your shoulders down.

GET IN POSITION: Begin by kneeling on the floor and sitting on your heels. Your feet should be comfortably together, with your knees apart and wider than your hips. Interlace your fingers in front of your chest and turn your palms away from your body. Extend your arms straight forward and up, reaching above your head, toward the ceiling. Lean back as you lengthen your abs and chest up and away from your hips. Continue to reach your arms up as you push your shoulders down. Maintain good posture and keep leaning back. (Avoid the temptation to lean forward.) Your head should be in line with your spine. Focus forward. Rock your arms side to side.

SERIES: 5-second hold (arms above head) 5-second hold (Lean arms right, ribs left.) 5-second hold (Lean arms left, ribs right.) 5-second hold (Hold arms above head and arch your back; tilt chin and focus eyes up.) 5-second hold (Reach arms out in front of your chest, push arms and palms out and away from you as you round your back.)

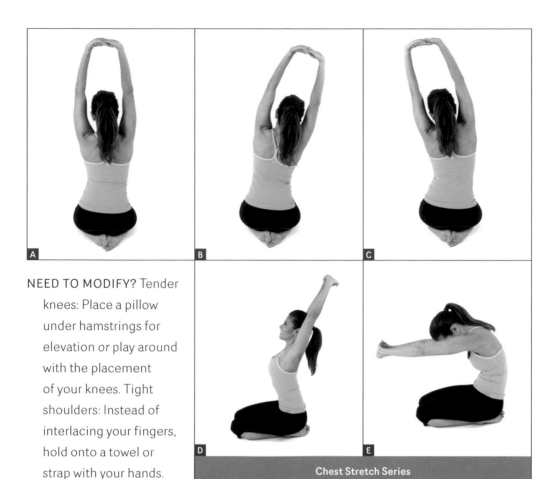

Chest Stretch Series

NEED TO MODIFY? Tender knees: Place a pillow under hamstrings for elevation *or* play around with the placement of your knees. Tight shoulders: Instead of interlacing your fingers, hold onto a towel or strap with your hands.

TRANSITION: Roll your body up and bring your legs out in front of you; flow into exercise 9.

9. Seated Leg Lift (Right)

FOCUS: Thighs

INTENTION: "I'm going to focus my energy on isolating my thigh."

GET IN POSITION: Begin by sitting on the floor with your spine perpendicular to your legs. Your right leg should be extended in front of you with your right foot flexed and your toes pointing up to the ceiling. Bend your left knee, sliding your left foot as close to your butt as possible. Interlace

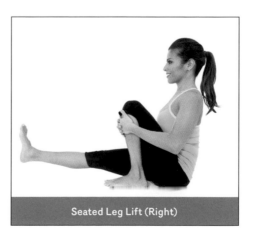

Seated Leg Lift (Right)

your fingers around your left knee and hug your leg in toward your chest. Engage your right thigh and lift your leg an inch off the floor, keeping your foot flexed. Keep your spine straight. Tighten your abs by pulling your belly button in toward your spine. Lift your abs and chest up and away from your hips. Keep your chest open, with your shoulders back and down, away from your ears. Keep your head in line with your spine. Focus forward.

GET MOVING: Ground your left foot into the floor and lift your right leg a couple of inches off the floor without involving your hip. Move your leg for the whole series without touching the floor, keeping your leg as straight as possible. Isolate your thigh. (Imagine a box sitting on top of your thigh that is being lifted up and down.) Maintain your posture and tap into your core strength. After the *bend/stretch* series, isolate your inner thigh by rotating your toes out to the right.

SERIES: 10 single count, *up/down* 10 pulses, *up/up* 10 single count, *bend/stretch* (Bend and lengthen your leg—make sure bends are tiny!) 10 single count, *up/down* (Turn your flexed right foot to the right, isolating your inner thigh.) 10 pulses, *up/up* (Keep your flexed right foot to the right, isolating your inner thigh.) 5-second hold (Turn your flexed right foot back to center.)

LOOK OUT FOR: Leaning too far back as a result of lifting your leg too high or not being aware of your posture. Not maintaining level hips. Swinging your leg instead of making deliberate movements. Touching your heel to the floor. Using your hip flexor instead of your thigh muscle to lift your leg.

NEED TO MODIFY? Feeling your hip flexor instead of your thigh: Bend your knee slightly and play around with the rotation of your leg. Tight back: Lean back slightly or sit on top of a block or pillow.

TRANSITION: Straighten out your left leg; bend and tuck your right leg as you lie back; flow into exercise 10.

10. Lying Thigh Stretch (Right)

FOCUS: Thigh

BREATHING TECHNIQUE: Inhale and squeeze your butt and hips up/Exhale and lean back as you lower your upper body.

GET IN POSITION: Begin in a seated position with your right foot under your right hip and your left leg extended in front of you.

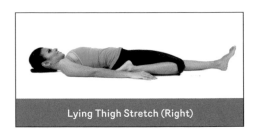

Lying Thigh Stretch (Right)

(Depending on how your knee feels, you may choose to place your right foot to the right side of your hips.) Your right toes should be behind your right heel. Keep your left foot flexed and in line with your left hip. Lean back until you are resting on your forearms. Your elbows should be in line with your shoulders. Keep your arms parallel, with your palms flat and fingertips spread. (If possible, lie completely flat on the floor.) Your hips should be squared. Squeeze your butt forward as you lean your upper body back. Keep your shoulders down. Focus forward.

SERIES: 10-second hold

NEED TO MODIFY? Tender knees: Lie down on your left side. Bend your right knee, take your right hand back, and grab your right foot. Bend your right elbow and pull your foot closer to your butt.

TRANSITION: Shift your weight back to sit and swing your right leg forward; flow into exercise 11.

11. Seated Leg Lift (Left)

Repeat exercise 9 with your left leg forward.

TRANSITION: Straighten out your right leg; bend and tuck your left leg as you lie back; flow into exercise 12.

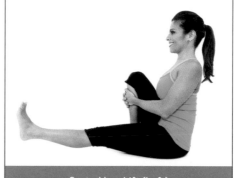

Seated Leg Lift (Left)

12. Lying Thigh Stretch (Left)

Repeat exercise 10 with your left leg back.

TRANSITION: Swing your left leg forward, straighten it, and lie on your back; flow into exercise 13.

13. Frog

FOCUS: Inner thighs

INTENTION: "Go, me! I'm lying here targeting that forgotten spot on the body. Feels great!"

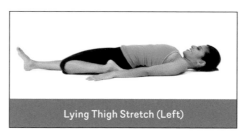

Lying Thigh Stretch (Left)

GET IN POSITION: Begin by lying flat on your back with your legs straight and perpendicular to the ceiling. Your arms should be resting by your sides. Place your feet in a V-shape, with your heels together and your toes apart. Keep your heels together as you bend your knees and lower your foot toward your butt. Spread your knees and thighs as wide as possible. (Think Plié.) Keep your heels together and in line with your tailbone.

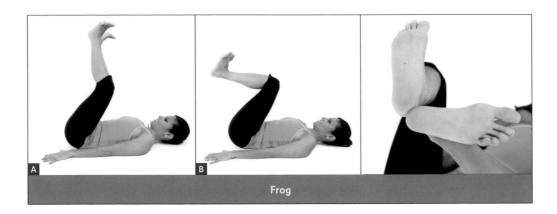

Frog

GET MOVING: Bend your knees, lower your feet toward your butt, and raise them back up to your original position. Keep your heels together! Imagine your heels are drawing a straight line up and down a wall. Continue to press your knees and thighs apart. (How far your knees can spread will depend on your hip flexibility.) Keep your back flat.

SERIES: 10 double count, *down/down/up/up* 10 single count, *down/up* 10 pulses, *up/up* 10 double count, *in/in/out/out* (Keep your heels together as you bring your knees and thighs together and then apart.) 10 single count, *in/out* (Keep your heels together as you bring your knees and thighs together and then apart.) 10 pulses, *out/out* (Keep your heels together and thighs apart and press your knees and thighs out and away from you—tiny movements, an inch in range.) 10 single count, *up/down*, full range 5-second hold (Bring your feet down as low as possible; press your knees out wide one last time.)

LOOK OUT FOR: Separating your heels. Dropping just your feet instead of opening and bending your knees wide enough that your feet naturally come down. Arching your back and not engaging and grounding your core.

NEED TO MODIFY? Tender hips: Do Seated Leg Lifts (p. 91) instead.

TRANSITION: Stay flat on your back, lower your feet to the floor; flow into exercise 14.

14. Inner Thigh Tucks

FOCUS: Glutes, hips, and inner thighs

INTENTION: "I can have fun right now."

GET IN POSITION: Begin by lying flat on your back. Bend your knees and draw your feet toward your butt, keeping your feet flat on the floor. Keep your feet, knees, and inner thighs together. (Squeeze your legs together so tightly it feels like you have one thigh.) Keep your toes in front of your heels.

GET MOVING: Engage your abs by pulling them in tightly and grounding your back into the floor. Tucking your pelvis under, press just your butt up and down off the floor (Try to find a good beat with your butt lifts, like you're bouncing a basketball.) Maintain a small range of motion. (Less is more!) Make sure to keep your abs engaged and your back flat as you isolate just your butt to lift your hips. You're flipping your hips up toward your chest, doing a mini-lift with your butt.

SERIES: 20 single count, *up/down* 20 single count, *up/down* knees apart (Keep your feet together; just open your knees.) 20 multi-count, *up/up/up/down* (Bring knees back together into original position.) 20 single count, *up/down* knees together (Keep your knees together; take feet apart.) 5-second hold

LOOK OUT FOR: Using your whole back to lift just your butt up. (Your back should not be off the floor.) Swinging your hips too high off the floor. Placing your feet too close to your butt. (Be nice to your knees!)

NEED TO MODIFY? Tender knees: Flex your feet or raise your heels instead of keeping your feet flat.

TRANSITION: Stay on the floor; flow into exercise 15.

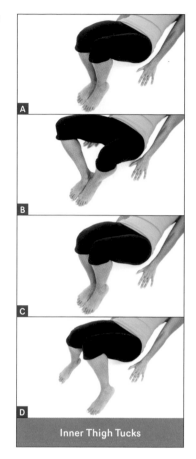

Inner Thigh Tucks

15. Lying Wide Straddle

FOCUS: Inner thighs and back

BREATHING TECHNIQUE: Inhale your chest up/Exhale and open your legs wider.

GET IN POSITION: Begin by lying flat on your back with your legs straight and perpendicular to the ceiling. Open your legs into a wide V. Place your hands on your inner thighs to support and spread your legs apart as far as your flexibility allows. Keep your legs straight and point your toes. Keep holding your legs as you circle your ankles/feet clockwise and counterclockwise.

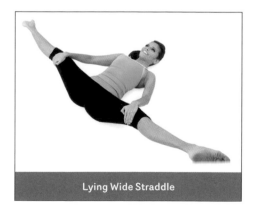

Lying Wide Straddle

SERIES: 5 single count, circles *ankles/feet clockwise* 5 single count, circles *ankles/feet counterclockwise*

NEED TO MODIFY? Tight groin or hips: Bend your knees slightly.

TRANSITION: Stay lying on the floor; flow into exercise 16.

16. Lying T-Stretch

FOCUS: Glutes

BREATHING TECHNIQUE: Inhale your knees into your chest/Exhale your lower back to floor.

GET IN POSITION: Begin by lying flat on your back with your knees bent and your feet flat on the floor. Cross your right leg over your left thigh, making sure there is no gap between your knees. Lift your left foot off the floor and bring your knees into your chest. Reach your arms up and forward and grab your ankles or shins. (Placement depends on flexibility and comfort.) Pull your knees and legs up toward your chest while pressing your butt down toward the floor. Pull your legs and feet apart while keeping your knees steady and pressing your hips down. Switch sides.

SERIES: 10-second hold, right side (right leg on top of left) 10-second hold, left side (left leg on top of right)

NEED TO MODIFY? Tight hips or back: Do Lying 4 Stretch (p. 185) instead.

TRANSITION: Lower your feet to the floor; flow into exercise 17.

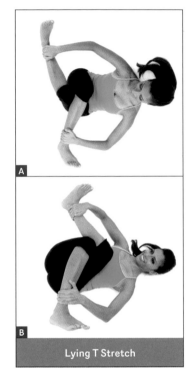

A

B

Lying T Stretch

17. Crunch Series

FOCUS: Core

INTENTION: "My focus will drive my strength."

GET IN POSITION: Begin by lying flat on your back. Bend your knees and draw your feet toward your butt, keeping your feet flat on the floor. Create a diamond shape with your legs by letting your knees fall open and placing the soles of your feet together in front of your groin. Move your feet either toward or away from you to find your "sweet spot." Clasp your hands and interlace your fingers behind your head. It should feel as if your head is resting on a "pillow" of your hands. Keep your elbows wide. (Note: Move through the series swiftly; don't take too long of a break between sets!)

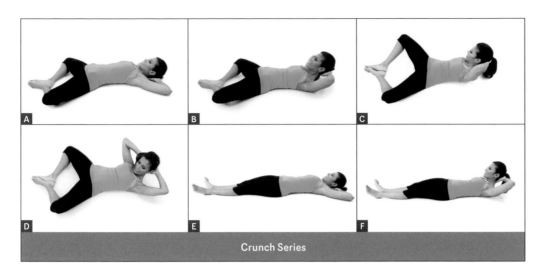

Crunch Series

GET MOVING: Curl your upper body up off the floor and "crunch" your abs. Come up high enough that your shoulder blades come off the floor. Keep your elbows wide. Make small movements. Keep your eyes focused on the ceiling.

SERIES: **Set 1:** *Diamond Crunch:* Keep your legs in a diamond shape and crunch your abs. 5-second hold, 20 single count, *up/down* 20 pulses, *up/up* 5-second hold (Hold last crunch.) Rest (a couple of seconds, not too long!) **Set 2:** *Diamond Twist Crunch:* Keep your legs in a diamond shape and crunch up toward your right and then your left sides. 5-second hold (Crunch body to the right, rotating left elbow to right slightly.) 20 single count, *up/down*, crunch to right 20 pulses, *up/up*, crunch to right 5-second hold (Hold last crunch.) Rest (a couple of seconds; not too long!) 5-second hold (Crunch body to the left, rotating right elbow to left slightly.) 20 single count, *up/down*, crunch to left 20 pulses, *up/up*, crunch to left 5-second hold (Hold last crunch.) Rest (a couple of seconds; not too long!) **Set 3:** *Straight Leg Crunch:* Stay flat on your back and extend your legs straight. Bring your feet into a V-shape with your heels together and your toes apart. Flex your feet. Keep your legs straight and crunch your abs. 5-second hold, 20 single count, *up/down* 20 pulses, *up/up* 5-second hold (Hold last crunch.) Rest (a couple of seconds; not too long!)

LOOK OUT FOR: Lifting your neck instead of your shoulders. Folding your elbows into your face instead of keeping them wide. Not curling up high enough. Not following a fast enough tempo.

NEED TO MODIFY? Tender neck: Keep your range small and rest your head into your hands even more.

TRANSITION: Flip over, flow into exercise 18.

18. Cobra

FOCUS: Core and back

BREATHING TECHNIQUE: Inhale your chest up/Exhale your hips forward and shoulders back.

GET IN POSITION: Begin by lying on your stomach, propped on your forearms. Slide your hands back under your shoulders, keeping your palms flat and fingertips spread. Keep your elbows bent, hugging them tightly into your body. Keep your feet and knees hip-width apart. Press the tops

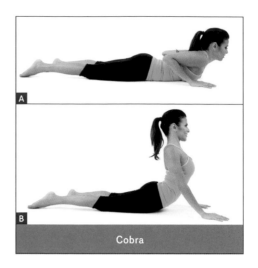

Cobra

of your feet, thighs, and hips firmly into the floor. Start to lengthen and straighten your arms while lifting your chest off the floor. Keep your shoulder blades back, puffing your ribs forward. Keep your hips connected to the floor and lift your upper body. (You might not be able to straighten your arms entirely, so feel free to keep your elbows slightly bent for comfort.) Firm up your butt and drive your hips forward while lifting your chest and stretching your abs. Twist your upper body to the right and to the left, lengthening your sides, and then return to center. (Repeat the movement twice.)

SERIES: 10-second hold

NEED TO MODIFY? Tender back: Do Cat/Cow (p. 99) instead.

TRANSITION: Lower your upper body; flow into exercise 19.

19. Superman Builder

FOCUS: Back

INTENTION: "I'm creating a stronger back. My posture will be better."

GET IN POSITION: Begin by lying on your stomach, resting your forehead on your hands. Keep your feet and knees hip-width apart. Engage and straighten your legs as you point your toes. Stretch your arms forward a little wider than your shoulders. Keep a slight bend in your elbows. Your palms should be facing down. Tighten your abs by pulling your belly button in toward your spine. Your head should be slightly off the floor. Try to keep your head in line with your spine. (Don't crank your head up!) Focus on the floor.

GET MOVING: At first, keep your legs steady as you lift just the upper half of your body (your arms and chest) up and down, using your back/posture muscles. Squeeze your shoulder blades together as your chest rises. Then, rest your forehead on your hands and keep your upper half steady as you lift just the lower half of your body (your legs) up and down, using your butt/back/posture muscles. Squeeze your butt slightly as your legs rise. Finally, lift both halves of your body (your arms and legs) using your back/posture muscles.

SERIES: 20 single count, *up/down*, upper half only 5-second hold, upper half lifted 20 single count, *up/down*, lower half only 5-second hold, lower half lifted 20 single count, *up/down*, both upper and lower halves 5-second hold, both upper and lower halves lifted

LOOK OUT FOR: Lifting your head instead of your arms and stressing your neck muscles. Not lifting your chest and legs high enough on the rise. Placing your feet too far apart. Forgetting to target your back muscles.

NEED TO MODIFY? Tender back: Lift up and down in Cobra (p. 69) instead.

TRANSITION: Lift up and come onto your hands and knees; flow into exercise 20.

20. Cat/Cow

FOCUS: Core and back

BREATHING TECHNIQUE: Inhale fully into Cow/Exhale fully into Cat.

GET IN POSITION: Begin on all fours (on hands and knees) with your feet and knees hip-width apart. Your hands should be under your shoulders and your knees under your hips. Keep your hips squared. *Inhale into Cow:* Drop your belly and arch

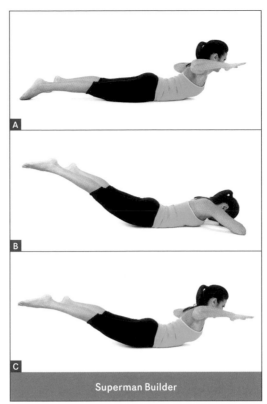

Superman Builder

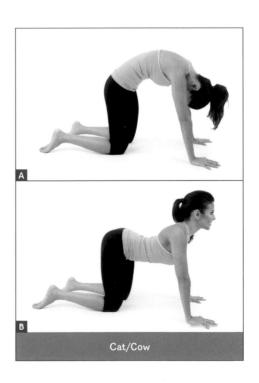

Cat/Cow

your back to bring your chest through your shoulders, moving your shoulders away from your ears. Your head and butt are reaching up toward the ceiling. *Exhale into Cat:* Round your back, drawing your belly up toward the ceiling. Drop your head toward the floor and tuck your hips.

SERIES: 3 breaths, *inhale/exhale* (3 Cows/3 Cats) Make sure to take full, long breaths.

NEED TO MODIFY? Tender knees: Fold your mat under your knees for extra cushioning. Tender neck: Avoid dropping your neck forward and pulling it back.

TRANSITION: Stay on your hands and knees; flow into exercise 21.

21. Down Dog

FOCUS: Hamstrings and back

BREATHING TECHNIQUE: Inhale your arms long and hips up/Exhale your shoulders down and heels toward the floor.

GET IN POSITION: Begin in Cat/Cow position, making sure your hands are slightly in front of your shoulders. Your palms (parallel or slightly turned out) should be flat

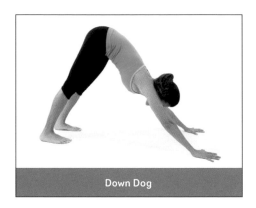

Down Dog

and your fingers spread. Curl your toes under and lift your knees and hips up. Start to shift your weight back and out of your shoulders. As you lengthen your arms and legs, continue to press your palms and heels down. As your hips rise toward the ceiling, push the tops of your thighs back and stretch your heels down to the floor, lengthening your hamstrings. Straighten your knees but do not lock them. Maintain straight legs. (Soften your knees if your lower back or hamstrings are tight.) Rotate your elbows in to firm up the arms and shoulders. Maintain a long back. Keep your head in line with your arms; do not hang your head down. (Note: Imagine you're creating a teepee with your body!)

SERIES: 10-second hold

NEED TO MODIFY? Tender knees or tight back and hamstrings: Keep your legs bent and heels raised.

TRANSITION: Walk your hands back toward your feet; flow into exercise 22.

22. Ragdoll

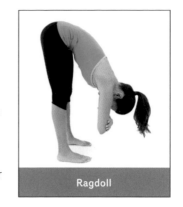

Ragdoll

FOCUS: Hamstrings

BREATHING TECHNIQUE: Inhale your hips up/Exhale your upper body toward the floor.

GET IN POSITION: Begin in Down Dog and walk your hands back toward your feet. Keep your feet parallel, with your toes in front of your heels. Grab hold of your elbows with your opposing hands. Maintain straight legs. (Soften your knees if your lower back or hamstrings are tight.) Keep folding your upper body over your legs, lengthening your spine. Hang, letting gravity pull your upper body toward the floor. Release any tension in your head and neck.

SERIES: 10-second hold

NEED TO MODIFY? Tight hamstrings or back: Keep your legs bent. (Don't pressure yourself to straighten your legs.)

TRANSITION: Roll your body up to stand; flow into exercise 23.

23. Standing Meditation

FOCUS: Total body awareness

MANTRA: Let go. Live. Love.

BREATHING TECHNIQUE: Inhale your chest up/Exhale your shoulders back.

GET IN POSITION: Begin by standing with your feet hip-width apart. Keep your feet parallel, with your toes in front of your heels. Maintain straight legs. Point your tailbone down. Tighten your abs by pulling your belly button in toward your spine. Stand tall as you lengthen your abs and chest up and away from your hips. Keep your chest open, with your shoulders back and down, away from your ears. Your head should be in line with your spine. Focus forward. Bring your palms together in front of your chest.

SERIES: 30-second hold or longer

NEED TO MODIFY? Close your eyes to help you focus better.

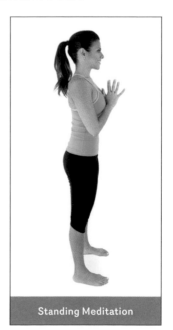

Standing Meditation

THE POST-WORKOUT

1 **Post-Workout Recap:**

Be proud of yourself. You transformed regular energy fuel into high-octane fuel through a productive and movement-filled workout.

Did my emotional weight change?

☐ YES ☐ NO

Did I accomplish my workout intention?

☐ YES ☐ NO

Is there a change in my physical body?

☐ YES ☐ NO

2 **My Post-Workout Mood Is:**

(Write down, think, or say out loud.)

_____

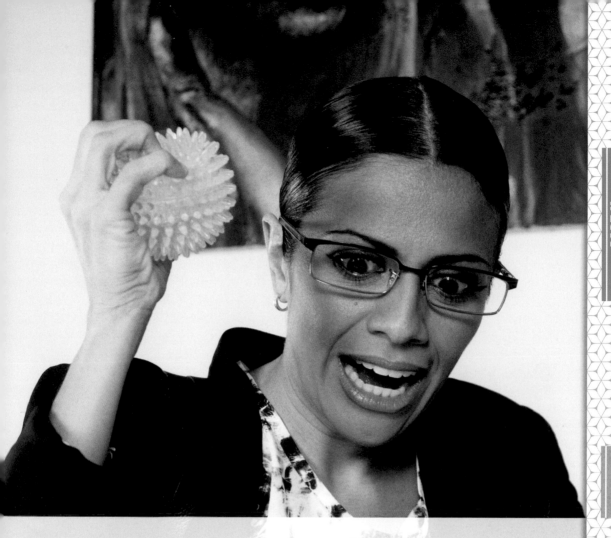

— CHAPTER 5 —

THE STRESS WORKOUT

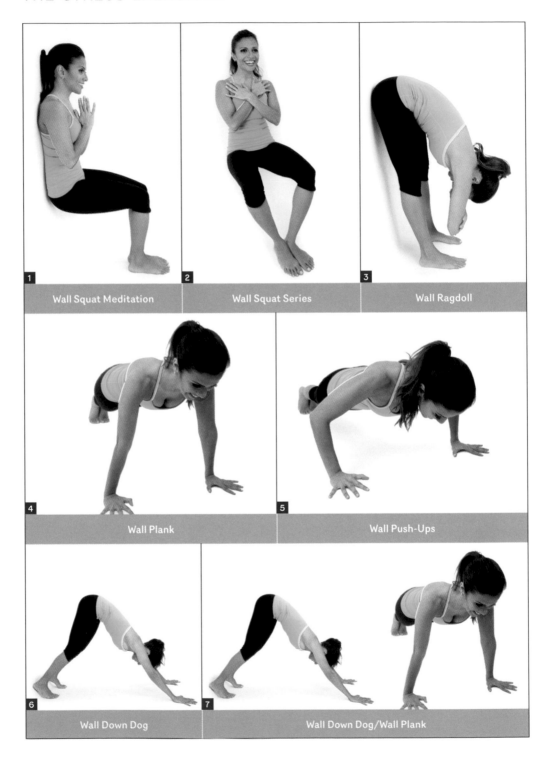

1. Wall Squat Meditation
2. Wall Squat Series
3. Wall Ragdoll
4. Wall Plank
5. Wall Push-Ups
6. Wall Down Dog
7. Wall Down Dog/Wall Plank

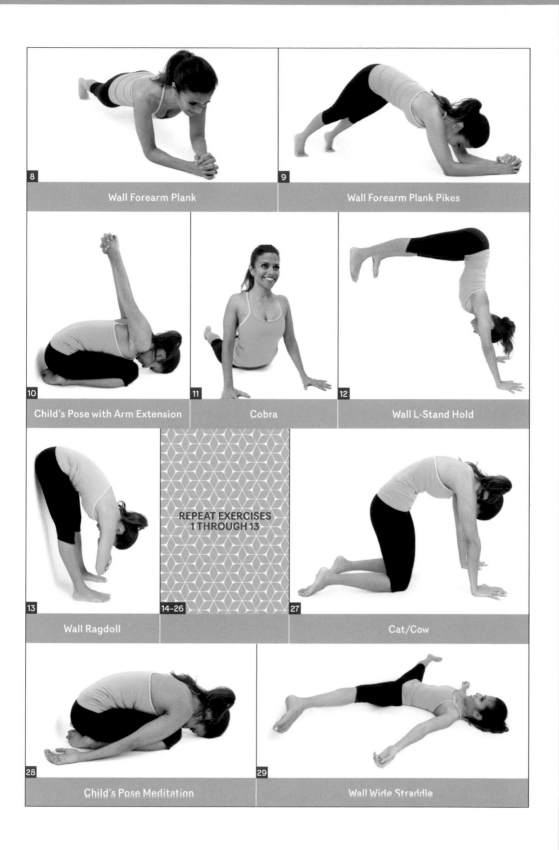

8 Wall Forearm Plank

9 Wall Forearm Plank Pikes

10 Child's Pose with Arm Extension

11 Cobra

12 Wall L-Stand Hold

13 Wall Ragdoll

14–26 REPEAT EXERCISES 1 THROUGH 13

27 Cat/Cow

28 Child's Pose Meditation

29 Wall Wide Straddle

W e have innate fight-or-flight responses to deal with stress—a mood that has the potential to take down even the strongest person.

There is such a huge range of everyday situations that leads us to stress: moving to a new city where you don't know anyone, ending a relationship, having a ton of work dumped on your desk on a Friday afternoon when you promised your kids you'd be taking them out to the park all weekend, even dyeing your hair the wrong color. And the kicker is that when you feel one stressor, within seconds it can quickly multiply. Sometimes stress can keep your mind so busy you don't know the problem is stress until you're lying in bed at night unable to sleep. That might turn into the moment you decide that you've finally reached your limit and something has got to give!

What is the emotional weight of all your stress and its resulting mood, and how is it manifesting in your physical body?

THE PRE-WORKOUT

1 **I Am Feeling:**

☐ Agitated	☐ Fearful	☐ Overburdened
☐ Angst	☐ Fretful	☐ Overwhelmed
☐ Annoyed	☐ Frustrated	☐ Pained
☐ Anxious	☐ Fussy	☐ Perturbed
☐ Apprehensive	☐ Grouchy	☐ Pressured
☐ Bothered	☐ Grumpy	☐ Provoked
☐ Careworn	☐ Harried	☐ Qualms
☐ Concerned	☐ Hassled	☐ Quarrelsome
☐ Confused	☐ High-Strung	☐ Resentful
☐ Crabby	☐ Hotheaded	☐ Shaken
☐ Cranky	☐ Impatient	☐ Strained
☐ Dejected	☐ Inadequate	☐ Stressed
☐ Demoralized	☐ Inconsistent	☐ Suspicious
☐ Depressed	☐ Irritable	☐ Tense
☐ Discomfited	☐ Jittery	☐ Tight
☐ Disquieted	☐ Misgivings	☐ Touchy
☐ Distressed	☐ Mistrustful	☐ Troubled
☐ Exasperated	☐ Nervous	☐ Uncertain

☐ Uncomfortable	☐ Unreliable	☐ Weird
☐ Uneasy	☐ Upset	☐ Worried
☐ Unnerved	☐ Vexed	

Choose from the list above, or add your own words. Then write down your mood *or* say it out loud and embrace it.

2 **My Current Mood Is:**

_____

3 **My Emotional Weight Is:**

1	5	10
Light	Neutral	Heavy

4 **My Physical Symptoms Are:**

☐ Aches and Pains	☐ Hand-Wringing	☐ Panic Attacks
☐ Acid Reflux	☐ Headaches	☐ Prickliness
☐ Adrenaline Rush	☐ Heartburn	☐ Rapid Breathing
☐ Agitation	☐ Heavy Breathing	☐ Rapid Heartbeat
☐ Binge Eating	☐ Heavy Chest	☐ Ringing in the Ear
☐ Chills	☐ Hunger	☐ Shaking
☐ Cold Palms and Feet	☐ Insomnia	☐ Stomachache
☐ Constipation	☐ Jaw Clenching	☐ Sweating
☐ Crying	☐ Jitteriness	☐ Teeth Grinding
☐ Cramps	☐ Low Energy	☐ Tightness
☐ Diarrhea	☐ Nail Biting	☐ Tingling
☐ Dizziness	☐ Nausea	
☐ Dry Mouth	☐ Nervousness	
☐ Goosebumps	☐ Pacing	

- I am so stressed out, I feel like I'm going to faint or get sick.

- This situation is never ever going to get better. I don't know if I can handle it anymore.

- It's due. Okay, okay . . . I've just got to suck it up and start.

- Am I still going to feel like this tomorrow?

- Are you kidding me?

- Why is this happening to me? I can't cope, I really can't.

- I know I'm eating mashed potatoes and chocolate pudding and Twizzlers for dinner, and I really don't care. I need to do *something* to make myself feel better.

- I can't sleep anymore. My mind is racing so much I can't stop thinking about what I have to deal with and I'm too crazed to sleep.

- I am *not* PMSing! Don't tell me I'm overreacting to my problems.

- I don't even have time to eat. There is not enough time in the day.

THE WORKOUT

1 **Mantra for Stress:**

Shut up. Sit. Smile.

Stress can either give me the kick I need to stop my procrastination right in its tracks, or kick my butt so hard the growing tension makes me wonder if I need to be tranquilized. All kidding aside, when this Type A woman is stressed-out, my training in yoga and breathing techniques feels like strange and impossible tools from a past life.

Numerous studies have shown over and over again how stress can leave you emotionally depleted and physically incapacitated. It's one of the reasons why people turn to self-medication and habits they know are unhealthy and self-destructive: the stress is so painful and can become so overwhelming that it can turn into a chronic condition with devastating results.

What's so amazing, however, about this whole stress mess is that stress can actually be healthy for you. After all, your bones need stress-bearing exercises, like Squats and Push-Ups, to remain strong. And your mind needs stress to remain sharp and tough.

The "Shut up. Sit. Smile" mantra is the stress-bearing exercise—the mental Push-Up—that can help manage your stress and emotional weight. It guarantees results; practicing it helps you become stronger and grow as an individual. It is hands down the hardest of my mom's mantras for me to live by. If you knew me, you would know that the phrase "shut up" doesn't sound like something I would say, let alone do. I rarely "sit," and I do "smile" easily, but never consciously.

We have all been in emotionally charged, stressful situations with people and things we care about. Whatever has been said and wherever the blame lies, anyone involved can benefit from my mom's simple mantra.

I was once in a relationship in which there was a lot of tension and hurt. Even though my boyfriend and I talked endlessly about our hopes, dreams, and frustrations, very little got resolved. When I despaired there was nothing I could do that I hadn't tried already and I felt like saying things that I would later regret, I remembered my mom's blunt mantra—and it worked! Forcing myself to shut up, sit, and smile allowed the tough moments to morph from tension to understanding. Giving myself the time to be quiet and listen helps me regain empathy and not butt in with unwelcome comments or advice. As a result, in tense situations (both personal and not) I can calm down and move forward.

This is all much easier said than done, of course. Sometimes life has to kick your butt to the curb for you to learn the value of a little meditation and a time-out. Stress can be a gift wrapped in some ugly paper. But unwrap it successfully and you will discover that what doesn't kill you truly makes you stronger.

One of my greatest challenges came about thanks to a couple of Indian peaches. When I was sixteen, during a highly coveted trip with my mom to her homeland, I ate two deliciously innocent-looking peaches that resulted in a life-threatening intestinal virus. This traumatic experience helped me gain insight into my mom's mantra, "Shut up. Sit. Smile."

Eating the peaches caused me to vomit uncontrollably and to lose weight very rapidly (I was already small, so this was scary) as well as my ability to walk. I hadn't spent much time in hospitals and had certainly never been in one filled with insects, lizards, and without running water. The doctors, who were confused by my symptoms, gave us mixed messages. I could get better or I could get worse. I spent long nights lying on cold hospital beds, warmed only by conversations with my mom and the kind nurses. My mom stayed with me day and night and I could see that she was scared I was going to die.

I thought that, too. Every day, my stress became as overwhelming as my ever-increasing need for human contact and for *life*. I didn't want to be lying there. It wasn't fair. I just wanted to see the Taj Mahal, eat spicy snacks, visit temples, and a hang with a few elephants!

Instead, my vacation became the time I spent with the comforting nurses and my sweet grandmother—they were my escape from the daily struggle. As we became closer, they began to represent healing and spirituality, and my feelings for them grew into an indestructible emotional strength that helped combat my fears. The bonds that developed were more fulfilling and powerful than any monument or temple I could have seen.

After four long and scary weeks in the hospital, the doctors cleared me to immediately board a plane to go back home. We returned to my uncle's house and I showered, put on fresh clothes, and prepared to go back to the hospital. I wanted to give the nurses my American CDs and other gifts to show them how much I appreciated and would miss them. I happily hopped into the car, but to my surprise, my mom said we were going straight to the airport. Given my fragile state, she thought I would get sick again if I went back. The pain of not saying goodbye to the nurses stressed me out even more than being sick. I thought my mom was being selfish and ungrateful, and I let rip some of the meanest things I've ever said to her, followed by the silent treatment. I later realized how unfair I'd been to my stressed-out mother who was saying goodbye to her family and preparing for a long flight home with an angry child who had just barely survived a month in the hospital.

Despite my appalling behavior, the only thing my ever-patient mom said was, "Rupa, I love you. This is in your best interest and your anger will eventually pass. Remember, if you shut up and sit, the smile will come." Not surprisingly, this made me even angrier. I already *was* shutting up, hoping to prove a point to my mom, and instead it was proving *her* point! I was sitting because I was still so weak that I had no choice, and I definitely couldn't see any of this trauma and stress resulting in a smile.

Before I embraced this mantra's lesson, the words *shut up*, *sit,* and *smile* were seemingly easy ones to understand. My mom's mantra, however, gave me a powerful tool for stress management and a priceless lesson in self-control and empathy.

Instead of "stop talking," my mom's definition of "shut up" was "turn off your mind chatter and your repetitive, debilitating thoughts, and cultivate your ability to listen."

Instead of "sit" being a position where your weight is supported by your butt rather than your feet, my mom's definition was "relax and release, and cultivate the feeling of being grounded."

Instead of "smile" being an amused facial expression, my mom's definition was "make something more pleasant and lighter."

So why didn't she just say, "Find some self-control, be present and listen, and eventually things will become lighter?" Because she knew it would feel fake. She knew I needed time to truly shut up, sit, and smile in order to manage my stress and to heal.

Sometimes it feels like stress is literally and figuratively impossible to survive. Whether it's your spouse or a stranger, the known or the unknown, somewhere underneath all that stress lie the gifts of this mantra's lesson.

If you can find the self-control and empathy to stay in the moment, your stress will begin to lighten, a solution will be made clear, and a genuine smile will start to surface naturally from within. The capacity to move forward and minimize stress has to do with quieting the noise in your mind, truly being in the moment, and listening. Sometimes you must force yourself to shut up and sit there, even though you're aching to move and speak. You must force yourself to be open even though you feel closed. This can be the quickest way to quieting the storm and attaining a sense of internal calm.

2 How to Use the Mantra

When people are stressed-out, they tend to be hypersensitive and overreactive. Couple that with feeling overwhelmed, and you can find yourself having no clue how to start tackling the stressful situation you are facing. In fact, unilaterally deciding on the definition of stress is stressing me out! But here it goes. Stress is more of a temporary situation that can be resolved through reflection guiding you toward balance. This is what differentiates stress from anger, which tends to come in short spurts and disappears once you process it and find means to get it out of your system. Stress also differs from anxiety, which is often connected to specific worries, sadness, or confusion and has a subconscious pattern of worry/stress-related thoughts often accompanied by physical reactions. Anxiety can surface in mild forms or be a diagnosable mental illness. And then there is doubt, which, although stressful, can usually be healed when you face it head-on and make an active commitment to seek courage beyond it.

"Shut up. Sit. Smile" is a healing tactic for stress. The centering and meditative nature of this mantra will create some space in your mind and allow room for the calm you're craving.

What you're looking for is balance, and the ability to tune out any strained mind chatter. Being in that heightened stress state always makes things worse than they are, especially when they truly are bad. That's where breath training and repetition of a mantra can be so helpful. "Shut up. Sit. Smile. Shut up. Sit. Smile." An even rhythm, breath, and focus have the power to center your thoughts and frenetic energy.

If you've ever meditated, it's likely that your first session wasn't easy, but if you are committed, focusing on breathing and repetition is actually an easy skill to master. Simply focusing on your breath will not only help you immediately in stressful situations, but also aid you with focus and regrouping in other areas of your life.

Having an accessible mantra like "Shut up. Sit. Smile" in your back pocket to use anytime and anywhere will help you feel confident that you can handle and combat the stressors thrown at you in life—because you know another butt kick *will* be coming!

3 Why the Stress Workout

By now you have taken the time to reflect on the source and scope of your stress and how it is weighing on you emotionally and physically. And if you're like me, it could weigh a *ton*!

The flow of this series is designed to lighten this weight while making you feel supported. You'll be doing most of the routine using a wall for support. You'll get additional support as the exercise sequence is repeated—that way, you don't have to stress about doing it perfectly the first time. Even better, its contemplative structure is specifically designed to help restore calm to your breathing and your entire being.

Embrace your mood, reflect on the mantra, and let it provide you with the incentive for a rejuvenating routine.

4 My Stress Workout Intention (Emotional or Physical) Is:

(Write down, think, or say out loud.)

MUSIC

Choose music that will soothe you and mitigate your stress. These tunes are easy on the ears, and have a good beat and hopeful choruses. Here are a few suggestions for songs that capture life's sometimes stressful journey well.

1960s: "Hey Jude" ▪ The Beatles
1970s: "Rhiannon" ▪ Fleetwood Mac
1980s: "Orinoco Flow" ▪ Enya
1990s: "Bittersweet Symphony" ▪ The Verve
2000s: "Snow (Hey Oh)" ▪ Red Hot Chili Peppers
2010s: "Anything Could Happen" ▪ Ellie Goulding

5 **The Stress Exercises**

Find an empty wall in a spacious area. Be sure you have enough space on either side and in front of you.

1. Wall Squat Meditation

FOCUS: Thighs and glutes

MANTRA: Shut up. Sit. Smile.

INTENTION: "I'm here. Let's do this. "

GET IN POSITION: Begin by standing and leaning back against the wall with your feet and knees together. Keep your feet parallel and a couple of feet in front of the wall, with your toes in front of your heels. Press your feet firmly into the floor. Slide down the wall until your hips are across from your knees, as if you are sitting in an invisible chair. (This is your squat position.) Keep your knees in line with your heels as you try to get your thighs parallel to the floor. Keep your tailbone down and your back completely flat. Press your feet down into the floor and lean your back into the wall to keep your body solid and secure. Tighten your abs by pulling your belly button in toward your spine. Keep your chest open, with your shoulders back and down, away form your ears. Your head should be in line with your spine. Focus forward. Bring your palms together in front of your chest.

GET MOVING: Put more pressure into your feet and lean your back against the wall. Tuck your tailbone under slightly, pressing your back into the wall. Maintain your posture and tap into your core strength.

SERIES: 1-minute hold

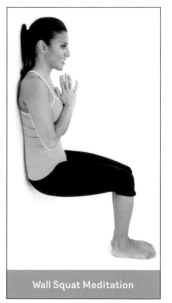

Wall Squat Meditation

LOOK OUT FOR: Sinking your butt too low or keeping it too high in the squat. Arching your back. Holding your breath. Tensing your shoulders. Forgetting to constantly ground your feet.

NEED TO MODIFY? Tender knees or back: Keep your hips up higher and don't bend your knees as much.

TRANSITION: Take a mini-break and then sink down again; flow into exercise 2.

2. Wall Squat Series

FOCUS: Thighs and glutes

INTENTION: "If I think I can do it, I can. I will try not to take a break."

GET IN POSITION: Begin by standing and leaning back against the wall with your feet and knees together. Keep your feet parallel and a couple of feet in front of the wall, with your toes in front of your heels. Press your feet firmly into the floor. Slide down the wall until your hips are across from your knees, as if you are sitting in an invisible chair. (This is your squat position.) Keep your knees in line with your heels as you try to get your thighs parallel to the floor. Keep your tailbone down and your back completely flat. Press your feet down into the floor more and lean your back into the wall to keep your body solid and secure. Tighten your abs by pulling your belly button in toward your spine. Keep your chest open, with your shoulders back and down, away from your ears. Your head should be in line with your spine. Focus forward. Cross your arms across your chest, making the letter *X*.

GET MOVING: Keep your back and head pressed against the wall and start to open and close your legs. Keep your feet grounded and together as you isolate your knees and thighs for movement. Tuck your hips under slightly. Press your feet firmly into the floor.

SERIES: 5-second hold 10 single count, *open/close* knees
5-second hold 10 single count, *open/close* knees
5-second hold 10 single count, *open/close* knees
5-second hold

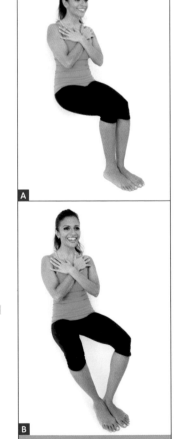

LOOK OUT FOR: Sinking your butt too low or keeping it too high in the squat. Arching your back. Holding your breath. Tensing your shoulders. Forgetting to constantly ground your feet. Rolling your feet out when opening and closing your legs. (You should isolate your knees and thighs only!)

NEED TO MODIFY? Tender knees or back: Stay up higher.

TRANSITION: Stand up, bend at your waist, and fold over; flow into exercise 3.

Wall Squat Series

3. Wall Ragdoll

FOCUS: Hamstrings

BREATHING TECHNIQUE: Inhale your hips up/Exhale your upper body toward the floor.

GET IN POSITION: Begin by standing against a wall with your butt touching the wall and your heels as close to it as possible. Keep your feet hip-width apart and parallel, with your toes in front of your heels. Reach your arms toward the floor as you fold your upper body over your legs, lengthening your spine. Grab hold of your elbows with your opposing hands. Maintain straight legs. (Soften your knees if your lower back or hamstrings are tight.) Hang, letting gravity pull your upper body toward the floor. Keep your butt pressed against the wall. Release any tension in your head and neck. Place your feet further away from or closer to the wall depending on your flexibility.

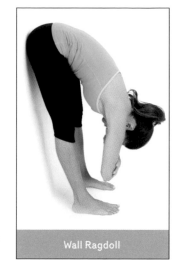

Wall Ragdoll

SERIES: 10-second hold

NEED TO MODIFY? Tight hamstrings or back: Keep your legs bent. (Don't pressure yourself to straighten your legs.)

TRANSITION: Place your hands on the floor and walk your body out; flow into exercise 4.

4. Wall Plank

FOCUS: Core and shoulders

INTENTION: "I can do this, stay calm, and focus on the form."

GET IN POSITION: Begin on all fours (on hands and knees) with your feet and knees together. Your hands should be in line with your shoulders, with your palms flat and fingertips spread. Curl your toes under, keep the balls of your feet flush to the wall, and press your heels back against the wall. Lift and straighten your legs. Level your hips and keep your back flat. Tighten your abs by pulling your belly button in

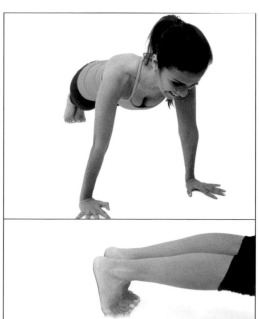

Wall Plank

toward your spine. Tuck your hips slightly so your back feels protected. Keep your chest open, with your shoulders back and down, away from your ears. Your head should be in line with your spine. Focus on the floor. Your entire body should feel solid, as if you're stuck in a tube. Continue to press your heels into the wall, as if you are about to break through it with your feet and body.

GET MOVING: Continue to monitor the flatness of your body. Push away from the floor while maintaining good posture. Maintain straight legs. Keep your chest open and your head in line with your spine. Keep shifting back and pressing your heels into the wall.

SERIES: 1-minute hold

LOOK OUT FOR: Keeping your hips too low or too high and arching or rounding your back as a result. Dropping your head. Rounding your shoulders. Placing your hands too close together or too far apart. Placing your hands too far forward and not in line with your shoulders. Arching your back instead of engaging your abs and tucking your hips slightly. Shifting your heels off the wall. (Note: Really use the wall! It's there for a reason!)

NEED TO MODIFY? Tender wrists or tight shoulders: Do Wall Forearm Plank (p. 121) instead. Tender back: Give yourself mini-breaks and be patient.

TRANSITION: Take a quick breather; flow into exercise 5.

5. Wall Push-Ups

FOCUS: Chest, arms, and core

INTENTION: "Even if it is tiny, it counts— and I'm getting stronger."

GET IN POSITION: Begin in Wall Plank position with your hands wider than your shoulders, palms flat and finger-tips spread. Keep your feet and thighs together. Straighten your legs. Keep the balls of your feet flush to the wall and press your heels against the wall. Level your hips and keep your back flat. Tighten your abs by pulling your belly button in toward your spine. Tuck your hips slightly so your back feels protect-ed. Keep your chest open, with your

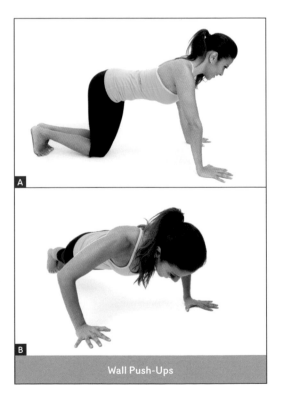

Wall Push-Ups

shoulders back and down, away from your ears. Your head should be in line with your spine. Focus on the floor. Your entire body should feel solid, as if you're stuck in a tube. Continue to press your heels into the wall, as if you are about to break through it with your feet and body.

GET MOVING: Bending your elbows and leading with your chest, lower your entire body down to the floor and then straighten your arms to lift your entire body back up. Lower yourself as far as you can without sacrificing your form—even a mini push-up counts! Make sure you keep pressing your heels back into the wall with every push-up. Maintain good posture and tap into your core strength for this workout.

SERIES: 20 single count, *down/up*

LOOK OUT FOR: Keeping your hips too low or too high and arching or rounding your back as a result. Dropping your head. Rounding your shoulders and not squeezing your shoulder blades together on the way down. Placing your hands too close together or too far apart. Placing your hands too far forward and not in line with your shoulders. Arching your back instead of engaging your abs and tucking your hips slightly. Taking your heels off the wall. (Use the wall!) Giving up because you can manage only a tiny range of movement.

NEED TO MODIFY? Tender wrists or tight shoulders: Make fists and substitute them for your flat palms. Tender back: Give yourself mini-breaks and be patient *or* do Push-Up Bent Knees (p. 88) instead.

TRANSITION: Shift your weight and hips back and up; flow into exercise 6.

6. Wall Down Dog

FOCUS: Hamstrings and back

BREATHING TECHNIQUE: Inhale your arms long and hips up/Exhale and ground your heels against the wall and toward the floor.

GET IN POSITION: Beginning in Wall Plank position, make sure your hands are slightly in front of your shoulders. Place your feet hip-width apart and parallel. Your palms (parallel or slightly turned out) should be flat and your fingers spread. Keep your toes curled as you shift your weight back (keep your heels against the wall, but the balls

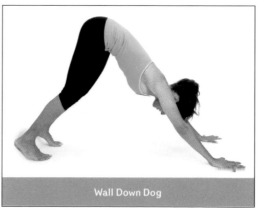

Wall Down Dog

of your feet can be a couple of inches away from the wall) and lift your hips up toward the ceiling. As you start to lengthen your arms and legs, continue to press your palms and heels down. As your hips rise toward the ceiling, push the tops of your thighs back and stretch your heels down to the floor, lengthening your hamstrings. Straighten your knees but do not lock them. Maintain straight legs. (Soften your knees if your lower back or hamstrings are tight.) Rotate your elbows in to firm up the arms and shoulders. Maintain a long back. Keep your head in line with your arms; do not hang your head down. (Note: Imagine you're creating a teepee with your body!)

SERIES: 10-second hold

NEED TO MODIFY? Tender knees or tight back and hamstrings: Keep your legs bent and heels raised.

TRANSITION: Shift your weight forward; flow into exercise 7.

7. Wall Down Dog/Wall Plank

FOCUS: Core, shoulders, back, and hamstrings

INTENTION: "I can enjoy my body and this moment."

GET IN POSITION: Alternate between Wall Down Dog and Wall Plank. Maintain good posture and tap into your core strength for this workout.

GET MOVING: Shift back and forth from Wall Down Dog to Wall Plank seamlessly, keeping your feet hip-width apart. Keep your legs straight. Keep your chest open, with your shoulders back and down, away from your ears. Your head should be in line with your spine. Keep your hands pressed firmly into the floor. Keep your heels pressed into the wall.

SERIES: 10 single count pikes *up/down* 10-second hold (in Wall Plank)

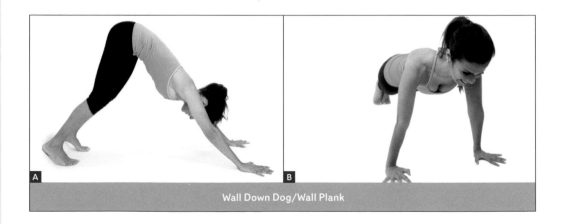

Wall Down Dog/Wall Plank

LOOK OUT FOR: Swinging your body instead of moving with control. Keeping your hips too low or too high and arching or rounding your back as a result. Dropping your head. Rounding your shoulders and not squeezing your shoulder blades together on the way down. Placing your hands too close together or too far apart. Placing your hands too far forward and not in line with your shoulders. Arching your back instead of engaging your abs and tucking your hips slightly. Using momentum or arm strength instead of using your core strength. Taking your heels off the wall. (Use the wall!)

NEED TO MODIFY? Tender wrists or tight shoulders: Do Wall Forearm Plank Pikes (p. 122) instead. Tender back: Give yourself mini-breaks and be patient.

TRANSITION: Shift your weight forward and drop to your forearms; flow into exercise 8.

8. Wall Forearm Plank

FOCUS: Core and shoulders

INTENTION: "I'm here; if I think I'm strong so will my body."

GET IN POSITION: Begin by lying on your stomach, propped on your forearms. Your elbows should be in line with your shoulders. Keep your feet hip-width apart. Clasp your hands together and interlace your fingers. Curl your toes under, keep the balls of your feet flush to the wall, and press your heels back against the wall. By pressing into your forearms and toes, lift your entire body off the floor. Level and adjust your hips to be in line with your shoulders, creating a flat back. Keep your legs straight. Tighten your abs by pulling your belly button in toward your spine. Tuck your hips slightly so your back feels protected. Keep your chest open, with your shoulders back and down, away from your ears. Your head should be in line with your spine. Focus on the floor. Your entire body should feel solid, as if you're stuck in a tube. Continue to press your heels into the wall, as if you are about to break through it with your feet and body.

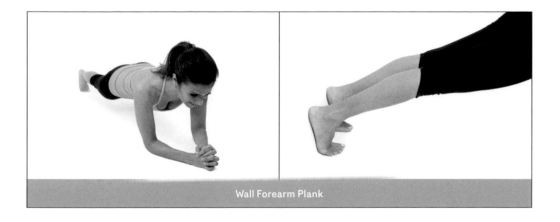

Wall Forearm Plank

GET MOVING: Continue to monitor the flatness of your body. Push away from the floor while maintaining good posture. Maintain straight legs. Keep your chest open and your head in line with your spine. Keep shifting back and pressing your heels into the wall.

SERIES: 1-minute hold

LOOK OUT FOR: Keeping your hips too low or too high and arching or rounding your back as a result. Dropping your head. Rounding your shoulders. Sticking your butt up instead of engaging your abs and keeping a flat back. Arching your back instead of engaging your abs and tucking your hips slightly. Forgetting to maintain strong legs. Shifting your heels off the wall. (Note: Really use the wall! It's there for a reason!)

NEED TO MODIFY? Tender back: Give yourself mini-breaks and be patient *or* do Wall Plank (p. 117) instead.

TRANSITION: Shift your weight back and hips up; flow into exercise 9.

9. Wall Forearm Plank Pikes

FOCUS: Core, shoulders, back, and hamstrings

INTENTION: "My core concentration will make this super-effective and safe."

GET IN POSITION: Begin in Wall Forearm Plank. Start to pike your hips up toward the ceiling and down seamlessly. Think of shifting into Wall Down Dog, but on your forearms, and then going back into Wall Forearm Plank. Maintain good posture and tap into your core strength for this workout.

GET MOVING: Shift your weight out of your shoulders up toward the ceiling, making a teepee with your body. Keep your legs straight. Keep your chest open, with your shoulders back and down, away from your ears. Your head should be in line with your spine. Keep your hands pressed firmly into the floor. Keep your heels pressed into the wall.

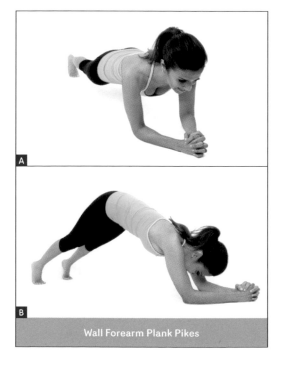

A

B

Wall Forearm Plank Pikes

SERIES: 10 single count pikes *up/down*
10-second hold (in Wall Forearm Plank)

LOOK OUT FOR: Swinging your body instead of moving with control. Keeping your hips too low or too high and arching or rounding your back as a result. Dropping your head. Rounding your shoulders and not squeezing your shoulder blades together on the way down. Placing your hands too close together or too far apart. Placing your hands too far forward and not in line with your shoulders. Arching your back instead of engaging your abs and tucking your hips slightly. Using momentum or arm strength instead of using your core strength. Taking your heels off the wall. (Use the wall!)

NEED TO MODIFY? Tender back: Give yourself mini-breaks and be patient *or* do Wall Down Dog/Wall Plank (p. 120) instead.

TRANSITION: Shift your weight and rest back; flow into exercise 10.

10. Child's Pose with Arm Extension

FOCUS: Shoulders and chest

BREATHING TECHNIQUE: Inhale your arms up and forward toward head/Exhale your lower back and hips down.

GET IN POSITION: Begin by kneeling on the floor and sitting on your heels. Your feet should be comfortably together, with your knees apart and wider than your hips. Fold your upper body forward between your thighs and bring your forehead to the floor. Clasp your hands together behind your back and reach your arms straight up toward the ceiling and forward toward your head. Rock your arms from side to side.

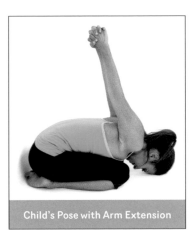

Child's Pose with Arm Extension

SERIES: 10-second hold

NEED TO MODIFY? Tender knees: Place a pillow under your hamstrings for elevation *or* play around with the placement of your knees until you feel comfortable.

TRANSITION: Using your arms and hands to slide your body forward, flow into exercise 11.

11. Cobra

FOCUS: Core and back

BREATHING TECHNIQUE: Inhale your chest up/Exhale your hips forward and shoulders back.

GET IN POSITION: Begin by lying on your stomach, propped on your forearms. Slide your hands back under your shoulders, keeping your palms flat and fingertips spread.

Keep your elbows bent, hugging them tightly into your body. Keep your feet and knees hip-width apart. Press the tops of your feet, thighs, and hips firmly into the floor. Start to lengthen and straighten your arms while lifting

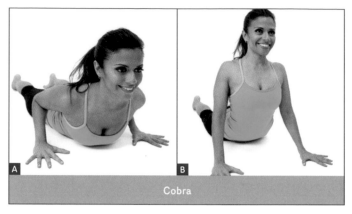

Cobra

your chest off the floor. Keep your shoulder blades back, puffing your ribs forward. Keep your hips connected to the floor and lift your upper body. (You might not be able to straighten your arms entirely, so feel free to keep your elbows slightly bent for comfort.) Firm up your butt and drive your hips forward while lifting your chest and stretching your abs. Twist your upper body to the right and to the left, lengthening your sides, and then return to center. (Repeat the movement twice.)

SERIES: 10-second hold

NEED TO MODIFY? Tender back: Do Cat/Cow (p. 125) instead.

TRANSITION: Lower your upper body, curl toes under, and push your weight back up; flow into exercise 12.

12. Wall L-Stand Hold

FOCUS: Back, shoulders, arms, core, and balance

BREATHING TECHNIQUE: Inhale your legs up/Exhale and ground your hands into the floor and feet into the wall.

GET IN POSITION: From a Wall Down Dog start to walk your feet up the wall. (Adjust your hand placement accordingly.) (Note: This takes practice; be patient as you get more comfortable with being inverted.) Walk your feet up the wall until your legs are parallel to the floor. Your body should form a 90-degree angle. Keep your feet in line with your hips and your hips in line with your

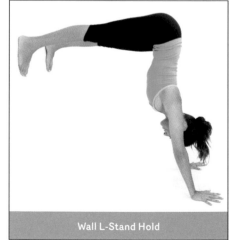

Wall L-Stand Hold

shoulders and palms. Continue to press your feet firmly back into the wall and your palms down into the floor.

SERIES: 20-second to 1-minute hold (depending on your comfort level)

NEED TO MODIFY? Tender wrists or tight shoulders: Begin from Wall Forearm Plank (p. 121) instead. Just a little fearful: Be patient, try to be a little more adventurous every time, *or* do Wall Ragdoll (p. 117) instead.

TRANSITION: Slowly lower your legs/feet down off of the wall and walk your arms back; flow into exercise 13.

13. Wall Ragdoll

Repeat exercise 3.

TRANSITION: Roll yourself up to stand; flow into exercise 14.

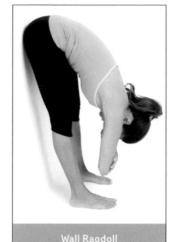

Wall Ragdoll

14–26. REPEAT EXERCISES 1–13.

(Note: That's right! You're doing it all again. This time you'll be even calmer because you'll know what to expect—you got this!)

TRANSITION: Come down to the floor onto all fours; flow into exercise 27.

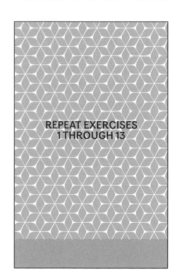

REPEAT EXERCISES 1 THROUGH 13

27. Cat/Cow

FOCUS: Core and back

BREATHING TECHNIQUE: Inhale fully into Cow/Exhale fully into Cat.

GET IN POSITION: Begin on all fours (on hands and knees) with your feet and knees hip-width apart. Your hands should be under your shoulders and your knees under your hips. Keep your hips squared. *Inhale into Cow:* Drop your belly and arch your back to bring your chest through your shoulders, moving your shoulders away from your ears. Your head and butt are reaching up toward the ceiling. *Exhale into Cat:* Round your back, drawing your belly up toward the ceiling. Drop your head toward the floor and tuck your hips.

SERIES: 3 breaths *inhale/exhale* (3 Cows/3 Cats) Make sure to take full, long breaths.

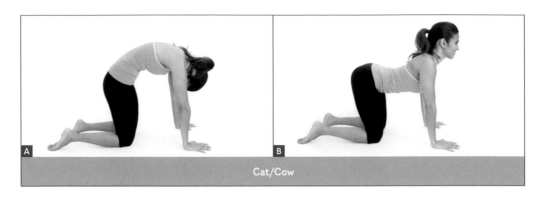

Cat/Cow

NEED TO MODIFY? Tender knees: Fold your mat under your knees for extra cushioning. Tender neck: Avoid dropping your neck forward and pulling it back.

TRANSITION: Shift your weight and rest back; flow into exercise 28.

28. Child's Pose Meditation

FOCUS: Shoulders and back

MANTRA: Shut up. Sit. Smile.

BREATHING TECHNIQUE: Inhale and exhale; observe your chest rising and falling. Embrace a sense of calm.

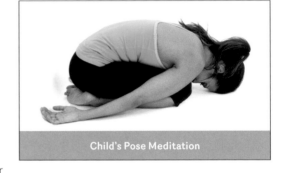

Child's Pose Meditation

GET IN POSITION: Begin by kneeling on the floor and sitting on your heels. Your feet should be comfortably together, with your knees apart and wider than your hips. Fold your upper body forward between your thighs and bring your forehead to the floor. Place your straight arms back alongside your torso with your palms up. Release your shoulders toward the floor.

SERIES: 10-second hold

NEED TO MODIFY? Tender knees: Place a pillow under your hamstrings for elevation *or* play around with the placement of your knees until you feel comfortable.

TRANSITION: Roll up and turn around toward the wall; flow into exercise 29.

29. Wall Wide Straddle

FOCUS: Inner thighs and back

MANTRA: Shut up. Sit. Smile.

BREATHING TECHNIQUE: Inhale your chest up/Exhale and ground your back and legs down. Embrace your patience.

GET IN POSITION: Begin by sitting with the right side of your body against the wall. With one swift movement, swing your legs up onto the wall and lay your shoulders and head onto the floor. (Note: It takes a bit of practice to find your rhythm here.) Try to have your butt flush with the wall, with your legs straight and perpendicular to the ceiling. Open your legs into a wide V. While pushing and inching your butt closer to the wall and inching your legs down into a wider V, spread your legs apart as far as your flexibility allows. Keep your heels pressed to the wall and your knees parallel and facing toward you; point your toes. You should feel comfortable as the weight of your legs settles down toward the floor.

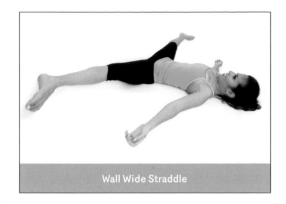

Wall Wide Straddle

SERIES: 1-minute hold (or even up to 5 minutes! Good for you if you can!) Be mindful and patient when coming out of this position. Bend one knee at time to carefully turn to one side and rest for a couple of moments before rising up.

NEED TO MODIFY? Tight groin or hips: Keep your butt farther away from the wall *or* maintain a small V.

THE POST-WORKOUT

1 Post-Workout Recap:

Be proud of yourself. You took your stress and managed it instead of letting it manage you. You forced yourself to quiet your mind and calm yourself for an invigorating workout.

Did my emotional weight change?

☐ YES   ☐ NO

Did I accomplish my workout intention?

☐ YES   ☐ NO

Is there a change in my physical body?

☐ YES   ☐ NO

2 My Post-Workout Mood Is:

(Write down, think, or say out loud.)

_____

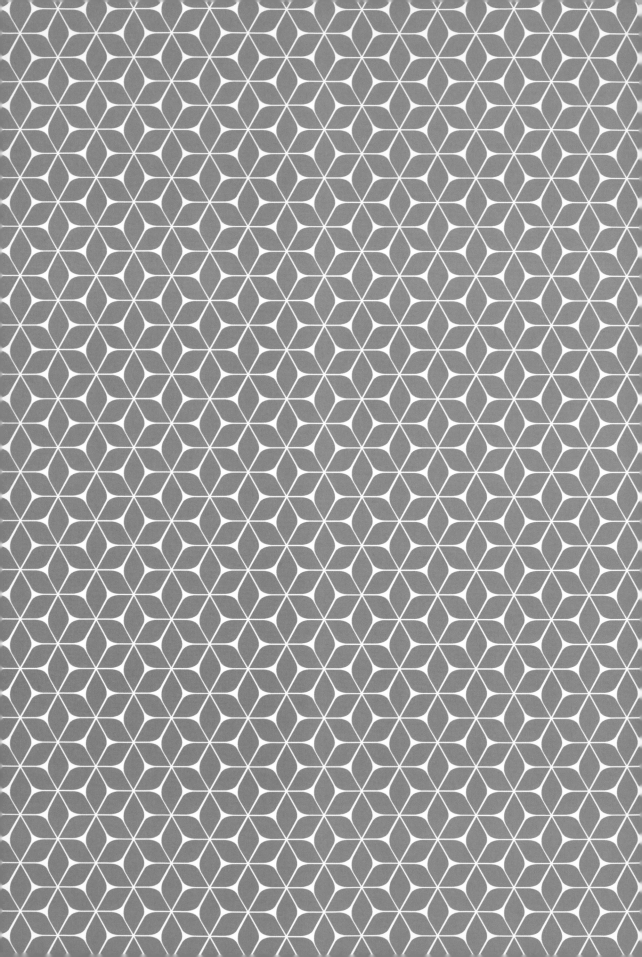

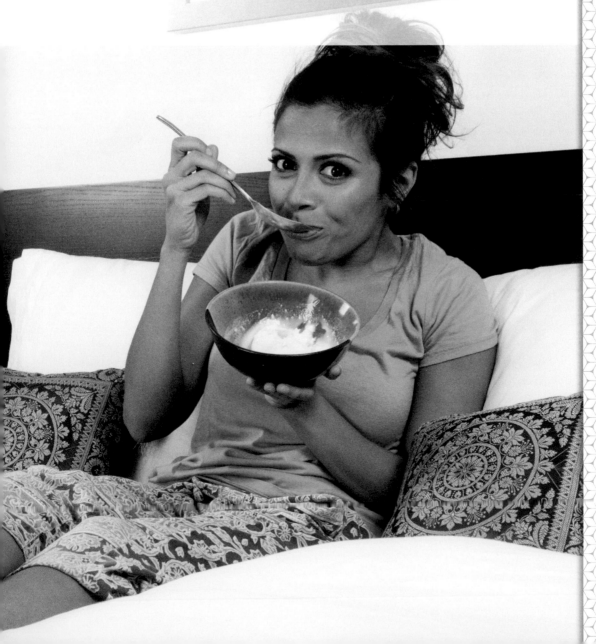

CHAPTER 6
THE CHILL WORKOUT

THE CHILL EXERCISES

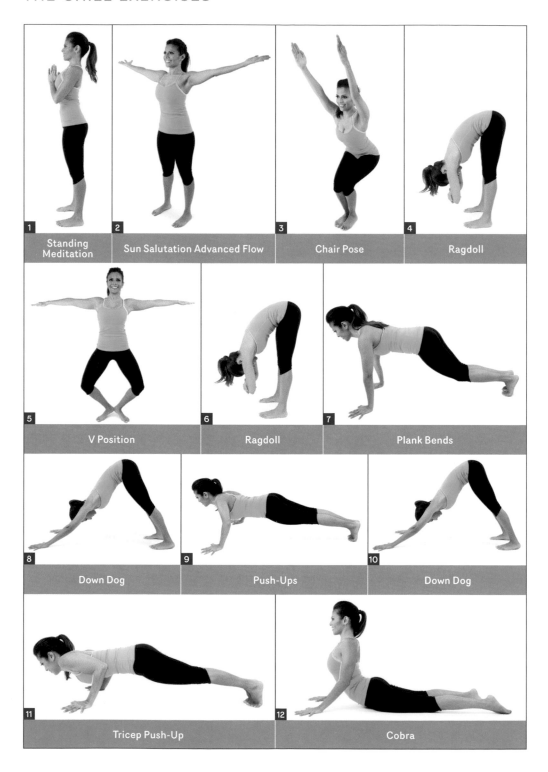

1. Standing Meditation
2. Sun Salutation Advanced Flow
3. Chair Pose
4. Ragdoll
5. V Position
6. Ragdoll
7. Plank Bends
8. Down Dog
9. Push-Ups
10. Down Dog
11. Tricep Push-Up
12. Cobra

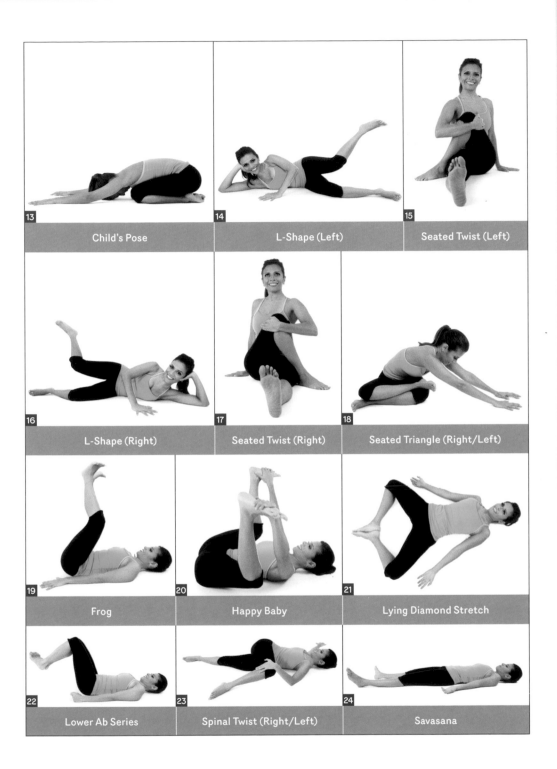

13 Child's Pose	**14** L-Shape (Left)	**15** Seated Twist (Left)
16 L-Shape (Right)	**17** Seated Twist (Right)	**18** Seated Triangle (Right/Left)
19 Frog	**20** Happy Baby	**21** Lying Diamond Stretch
22 Lower Ab Series	**23** Spinal Twist (Right/Left)	**24** Savasana

nlike the other six moods, chill is a mood that seamlessly reflects a calm and confident state of mind. No internal fight, no need to interpret a thought, no need to delve deeper. You are at peace with what you are. Whether you just peeled your bikinied self out of a hammock in the Caribbean or are having a lazy Sunday, about to watch your favorite TV series with the perfect iced tea in hand, there's no doubt here: You are tuned into that delicious zone of contentment.

The only thing to watch out for is that you can become so chill it might lead to a self-absorbed kind of laziness, with procrastination and even a bit of depression as a result. If you hear yourself saying, "I don't care, I'm all good, and that is kind of all that matters right now to me or anyone else," then it's time to pull yourself up out of the chill zone!

What is the emotional weight of your zone and its resulting mood, and how is it manifesting in your physical body?

THE PRE-WORKOUT

1 I Am Feeling:

☐ Acceptance	☐ Laid-Back	☐ Self-Indulgent
☐ Appreciative	☐ Lazy	☐ Selfish
☐ Calm	☐ Let Go	☐ Serene
☐ Complete	☐ Lightened Up	☐ Slowed Down
☐ Destressed	☐ Loosened Up	☐ Slothful
☐ Dismissive	☐ Nurturing	☐ Sluggish
☐ Dreamy	☐ Peaceful	☐ Still
☐ Embracing	☐ Procrastination	☐ Thankful
☐ Grateful	☐ Quiet	☐ Together
☐ Hungover	☐ Relaxed	☐ Tranquil
☐ Lackadaisical	☐ Released	☐ Unwound

Choose from the list above, or add your own words. Then write down your mood *or* say it out loud and embrace it.

2 **My Current Mood Is:**

_____

3 **My Emotional Weight Is:**

1	5	10
Light	Neutral	Heavy

4 **My Physical Symptoms Are:**

☐ Ability to Focus   ☐ Evenness   ☐ Muscle Relaxation

☐ Clarity   ☐ Increased Dopamine   ☐ Sense of Well-Being

☐ Easy Breathing   ☐ Increased Energy   ☐ Steadiness

☐ Easy Digestion   ☐ Increased Faith

☐ Endorphin Release   ☐ Lack of Nervousness

TEN COMMON **CHILL** THOUGHTS

- Could this day get any better? I don't think so.
- I feel so deliciously lazy, I think I'll stay in bed and watch trashy movies all day. I deserve it!
- I am just so calm and happy. Life is good.
- There's nothing better than taking some time for myself.
- I've been meaning to try that new massage oil/bath oil/scented candle/expensive perfume my mother bought me, and today is the day.
- Sure, you can come over and keep me company, as long as you don't expect me to go anywhere.
- I love the sound of rain and thunder when I'm all tucked in and cozy, safe from whatever's outside.
- You build the fire and I'll light it. Thanks!
- I put in a super-hard workweek; I deserve that extra glass of wine and a break.
- I'm kind of amazing. I wish every day was like today. I could do this forever.

THE WORKOUT

1 **Mantra for Chill:**

Love yourself dearly. Be yourself completely. Treat yourself occasionally.

I've been a New Yorker for over seventeen years, and I must say "I feel chill" may be the rarest sentence I hear or even say myself! It's something I strive for because being in a chill state of mind is a gift and a break from the daily routine and stressors we all have to face.

When feeling chill, you want to be in the moment and immerse yourself in appreciation of the mood. Wherever your vibe takes you, it's a special mood. It's that happy time when you're at peace with yourself and the world. You're relaxed, so you're not highly energized—and that's a good thing. We all need a break to lie back and not just smell the roses, but indulge in that bowl of double-fudge peanut butter ripple ice cream. (And not feel guilty about it either!)

We often want the high of feeling chill to last days, weeks, months, years . . . I mean, why not? But we all know that's not the way of life (nor should it be), so when this wonderful mood comes around, embrace it and enjoy it because it's a special treat. Your stay at Hotel Chill won't last forever, so when you've checked in, bask in it!

The "Love yourself dearly. Be yourself completely. Treat yourself occasionally" mantra is a means of increasing the pleasure of your mood and planting seeds for you to stay at Hotel Chill again in the near future.

It's ironic, but I learned the value of this mantra after an intense relationship with a wonderful man. We had tried everything—communication, therapy, vacation, time apart—that we thought could lower the unhealthy level of extremity upon which the relationship was founded. But nothing worked. We just never seemed to be able to chill together, to relax individually or as a team—which, for me, is an essential component of any thriving relationship. Being able to hang loose and be utterly comfortable with myself and my partner is as important as being able to set goals for myself and work hard toward them.

So we went through a gut-wrenching yet amicable and respectful breakup. I came to this pivotal decision after a long and emotional internal struggle. I had loved this man immensely for three years and dreamed of having a future with him, but my true spirit did not want to be in the relationship.

About six months before the relationship ended, my boyfriend and I were spending the weekend with my family and everybody seemed to be enjoying the time together. But he and I had been fighting more and more and I found myself hiding behind closed doors much of the time, desperately craving a chill life with zero fights and stress. That was when my mom and I had one of those all-important conversations.

"Rupa, if you get married one day and you are struggling and feel in your heart it isn't working, don't worry too much," she told me one morning. "And, if I'm not around but you feel you need my approval or support to end it or get a divorce, you don't. We're in America now. You can do anything. I trust the way I raised you. You have the tools to love yourself and be happy. And I will always love you and give you advice while I'm here. I mean I *am* your mom! I love your boyfriend, but I love *you* more, and if you want advice on how to make it work or not work, let me know. But remember this: "Love yourself dearly. Be yourself completely. Treat yourself occasionally."

I had heard this mantra before but when my mom said it that day, she generously showed me that I could offer myself simplicity, insightfulness, and compassion. And that I could get myself back to that chill place I needed. I was at a point where I wanted to start the brave and liberating task of ending the relationship but I didn't know where to begin. My mom instinctively knew that I needed less self-questioning and more loving guidance.

Interestingly, whenever I am going through a difficult or easy time, I find great comfort in this mantra. It really helps click me toward the chill place I know I need to find or to enjoy the roots of the chill place I'm in. I feel like I'm in my mom's kitchen watching her lovingly put butter into everything (even as I beg her not to!). As I repeat the mantra, I feel like I'm giving myself a hug or taking the first step toward healing myself after a trying time. For me, the comfort in the mantra is in the adverbs. My mom's choice of the words *dearly*, *completely*, and *occasionally* truly grounds this powerful lesson in balance.

For her, *dearly* and *completely* have different meanings from their tradional definitions and serve different purposes. *Dearly* implies a fulfilling love that is wholehearted but comes at an essential cost: embracing and owning up to your role in your own life, including your flaws and mistakes. This means taking responsibility for your actions, apologizing when necessary, and saying thank you without an ego. When you own up to your life, you can allow your true self to be revealed entirely without hiding, blaming, being defensive, or feeling insecure. It's only when you love yourself *dearly* that you can be yourself *completely*—and be able to relax and chill out in the knowledge of who you are.

When I finally did decide to end the relationship, I kept asking myself if I had failed in some way. I wondered if I would ever fall in love again. My mom did not discourage me from asking the questions, but she encouraged me to think of her mantra as a unifying theme I could come back to. It helped me quiet the noise in my mind and truly connect again; I was able to love myself dearly, move back to my core—and as a result, chill.

When you make mistakes, it's much better to take responsibility, apologize, and move on with a pledge to do better in the future. Everything you do is reflective of you, and ultimately, you have the tools to love yourself *dearly* and be yourself *completely*. When you embrace this, the weight of life lessens and you'll feel taller and more confident—literally and figuratively. And since I'm an even five feet tall, a little extra height is always welcome!

Although the essence of being you *completely* is healthy and empowering, my mom believes it can be deceiving as well, overshadowing the rest of the mantra. The lesson in attaining and appreciating a chill mood is only complete when all three aspects are embraced equally, which is where "Treat yourself occasionally" fits in.

Again, my mom makes a clear distinction between *occasionally* and *completely*. Her concern is that you could get caught up in thinking that if you are yourself completely, you are allowed to *treat* yourself completely. So what's wrong with that? Well, if you only think of yourself—if you stay in a chill, blissful state all the time—you might be foolish and indulgent, justifying your actions with, "I deserve it, I earned it, and I want it." So, she taught me to treat myself *occasionally* in great moderation, not *completely*.

For me, "Treat yourself occasionally" is the cherry on top of this lesson. My mom always says, "Rupa, when your spirit is in need of a hug, it's nice to treat yourself. So go get some ice cream, a new pair of sneakers, or hang with your friends and play games. Go enjoy something full of pleasure. But Rupa, don't do it too much." Ultimately, being myself isn't using external sources of happiness to define myself, and if I focus too much on these external things, I lose the person I am on the inside. I am myself *completely* only when I am not sidetracked by the external and am able to turn my focus inward and find my true spirit.

Just because we deserve chill time doesn't mean it should happen all the time! After all, if you lived in a chill state all the time, it would no longer be special, would it?

When we tap into our inner spirit, we embrace and accept the parts we like as well as those we don't like, which builds our self-confidence. Having a healthy inward focus with a removed desire of the external is the essence of this mantra. "Love yourself dearly. Be yourself completely. Treat yourself occasionally" means letting your spirit shine through with no judgment or self-denigration, but with balanced reflection and self-control. This loving mantra allows you to chill and prolongs that chill when the perfect moment strikes.

That's when I slip into my M. C. Hammer pajama pants, grab my Hershey's chocolate syrup and slather it over vanilla ice cream, turn on reruns of *Law and Order,* and dream about my next vacation.

2 How to Use the Mantra

Bask in your emotional weight. Feel the gifts of chill. Yes, it may sound cheesy, but appreciate that internal smile your heart is sporting.

It's helpful to think of how this chill mood feels in your mind, body, and heart. Openly welcome your contented self—strengths, weaknesses, and all. Chill is the state of mind where there are no goals, no rules, no judgments, and no guilt. Revel in it! Treat yourself to a gratifying workout all about loving your physical and emotional self and being *you.*

Repeat the "Love yourself dearly. Be yourself completely. Treat yourself occasionally" mantra throughout the workout. Let it be the love you give your heart and body.

3 Why the Chill Workout

Isn't it great to be in that chill space? Even when you're super relaxed, you can still use this mood to do an incredible workout.

The flow of this exercise series is designed for you to tap into your wonderful blissed-out state of mind, as you will have the space to enjoy and be who you are in the moment. Your feelings are slowed down and tranquil, and your body feels the same. Whether after a long day in the sunshine at the beach with people you love, at a new stage in the relationship with your partner, or having a tiny bit of a hangover from a fabulous party you went to the night before, you can yawn, stretch, and relax. It's really okay to feel lazy, too. You deserve this treat.

Embrace your mood, reflect on the mantra, and let it provide you with the ease and patience to be present in this relaxing and loving routine.

4 My Chill Workout Intention (Emotional or Physical) Is:
(Write down, think, or say out loud.)

5 The Chill Exercises

1. Standing Meditation

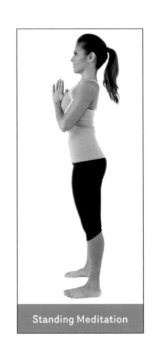

Standing Meditation

FOCUS: Total body awareness

MANTRA: Love yourself dearly. Be yourself completely. Treat yourself occasionally.

BREATHING TECHNIQUE: Inhale your chest up/Exhale your shoulders back.

GET IN POSITION: Begin by standing with your feet hip-width apart. Keep your feet parallel, with your toes in front of your heels. Maintain straight legs. Point your tailbone down. Tighten your abs by pulling your belly button in toward your spine. Stand tall as you lengthen your abs and chest up and away from your hips. Keep your chest open, with your shoulders back and down, away from your ears. Your head should be in line with your spine. Focus forward. Bring your palms together in front of your chest.

SERIES: 30-second hold or longer

NEED TO MODIFY? Close your eyes to help you focus better.

TRANSITION: Stay right there; flow into exercise 2.

2. Sun Salutation Advanced Flow

FOCUS: Total body strength and flexibility

INTENTION: "I'm going to enjoy discovering my body's flow."

GET IN POSITION: Be familiar with the Sun Salutation Basic Flow breakdown below. Breathing consciously is key to all Sun Salutations—make sure to take long, full breaths. Always link the motion of your breath to the movement of your body. The **bold-face instructions (Step 6)** indicate where the degree of difficulty will increase each time in the series and what will make this Basic Flow more "advanced." *Sun Salutation Basic Flow:* 1. Stand in Standing Meditation. 2. Sweep and raise your extended arms up toward the ceiling, palms facing and touching each other (inhale). 3. Turn your palms out, sweep your arms down, and bend at your waist into Standing Forward Bend (exhale). 4. Lift your upper body to a flat back (inhale). 5. Fold your body over again into Standing Forward Bend (exhale). 6. **Step back with your right leg and then your left leg, into Plank** (inhale). 7. Push into Down Dog; hold for 5 breaths (exhale). 8. Bend your right knee to step your right foot and then your left foot forward (inhale). 9. Adjust and try to flatten your palms against the floor in Standing Forward Bend (exhale). 10. Sweep and raise your extended arms up toward the ceiling, palms facing and touching each other (inhale). 11. Turn your palms out, sweep your arms down, and stand in Standing Meditation (exhale).

GET MOVING: Perform 3 Sun Salutations (from above) and increase the degree of difficulty each time by replacing **Step 6** with the direction from the series below.

SERIES: *Sun Salutation 1:* 1-minute hold in Plank *Sun Salutation 2:* 10 single count *bend/ stretch* in Plank and 10 single count push-ups *down/up* Sun Salutation 3:* 10 single count *bend/stretch/down/up* Push-Ups**

*Bend/stretch meaning: Maintaining a flat back, bend and stretch just your knees and then straighten your legs. Make sure your bends are tiny as you keep the rest of your body solid. **Think of it simply! You're combining the two different parts from Sun Salutation 2: bend and stretch your knees once and then perform a push-up by lowering and raising your body once. Repeat 10 times.

LOOK OUT FOR: Rushing and forgetting to link your breath to your flow. Putting pressure on yourself to demonstrate more flexibility and strength. (This is really all about flow!) Keeping your hips too low or too high and arching or rounding your back as a result. Dropping your head. Rounding your shoulders. Placing your hands too close together or too far apart. Placing your hands too far forward and not in line with your shoulders. Bending your knees too much and sacrificing the flatness of your back. Being bouncy

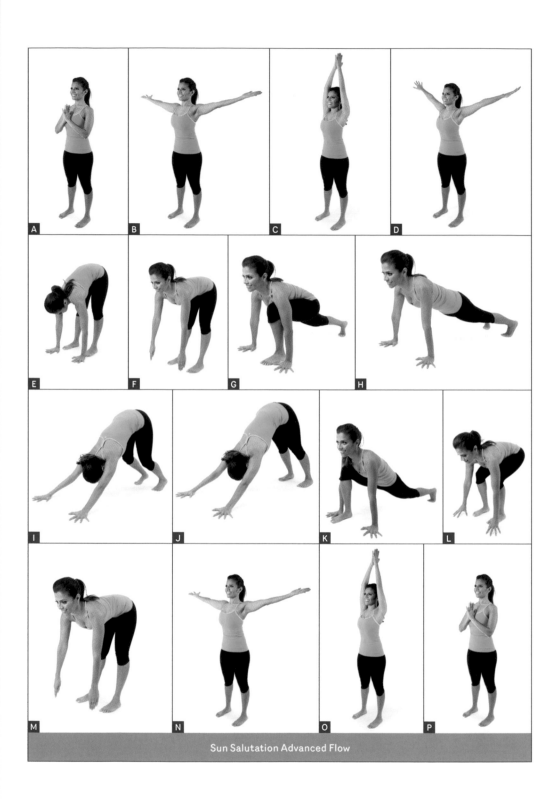

Sun Salutation Advanced Flow

in your movements instead of controlled. Arching your back instead of engaging your abs and tucking your hips slightly. Forgetting to tip your heels forward in Step 6.

NEED TO MODIFY? Tight hamstrings: Bend your knees in Standing Forward Bends. Too challenging: Slowly build as desired or stick with the Sun Salutation Basic Flow only.

TRANSITION: Reach your arms up and sink your body down; flow into exercise 3.

3. Chair Pose

FOCUS: Thighs, back, and glutes

BREATHING TECHNIQUE: Inhale your arms up/Exhale your hips down.

GET IN POSITION: Begin by standing with your feet and knees together. Keep your feet parallel, with your toes in front of your heels. Keep your knees in line with your heels as you bend your knees and drop your hips, trying to get your thighs parallel to the floor. Press your feet firmly into the floor. Lean forward slightly with your upper body until your back and thighs form a 90-degree angle. Keep your back flat and extend your arms straight up to the ceiling. Tighten your abs by pulling your belly button in toward your spine. Your arms should be parallel to your shoulders with your shoulders back and down, away from your ears. Face your palms toward one another and reach through your fingertips. Keep your tailbone down. Put more pressure on your heels, shifting your weight back. Your head should be in line with your spine. Focus forward.

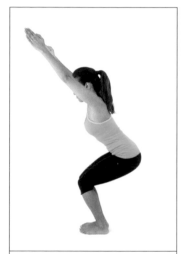

SERIES: 5 breaths, *inhale/exhale* 10 single count, *down/ up* (Keep your feet and knees steady as you move just your hips down and up.) 5 breaths, *inhale/exhale* Make sure to take full, long breaths.

NEED TO MODIFY? Tender knees or back: Keep your hips up higher.

TRANSITION: Fold your body over and walk your feet wider; flow into exercise 4.

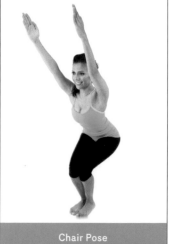

Chair Pose

4. Ragdoll

FOCUS: Hamstrings

BREATHING TECHNIQUE: Inhale your hips up/Exhale your upper body toward the floor.

GET IN POSITION: Begin by standing with your feet hip-width apart. Keep your feet parallel, with your toes in front of your heels. Reach your arms toward the floor as you fold your upper body over your legs, lengthening your spine. Grab hold of your elbows with your opposing hands. Maintain straight legs. (Soften your knees if your lower back or hamstrings are tight.) Hang, letting gravity pull your upper body toward the floor. Release any tension in your head and neck.

SERIES: 10-second hold

NEED TO MODIFY? Tight hamstrings or back: Keep your legs bent. (Don't pressure yourself to straighten your legs.)

TRANSITION: Lift your upper body up; flow into exercise 5.

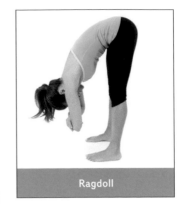

Ragdoll

5. V position

FOCUS: Thighs, calves, and glutes

INTENTION: "My poise can help sculpt strength and results."

GET IN POSITION: Begin by standing with your feet in a V-shape (heels together, toes apart). Lift your arms up and across from your shoulders, forming a T-shape. Keep your palms facing down. Bend both knees, keeping them in line with your toes. Drop your

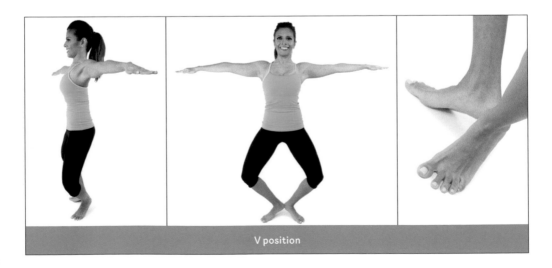

V position

hips down a couple of inches, keeping your butt in line with your heels and your shoulders in line with your hips. Keeping your heels together, lift your heels an inch off the floor. Point your tailbone down. Tighten your abs by pulling your belly button in toward your spine. Lift your abs and chest up and away from your hips. Keep your chest open, with your shoulders back and down, away from your ears. Keep your head in line with your spine. Focus forward.

GET MOVING: Keeping your feet steady, bend your knees as you lower your hips down and up. Pretend your back is sliding up and down an imaginary wall, as you keep leaning your upper body back. Make sure your heels stay raised and pressed together. Keep reaching through your fingertips as you lengthen your arms and keep them up and across from your shoulders.

SERIES: 5-second hold (hold at a range where you feel your strength being challenged) 10 single count, *down/up* 10 pulses, *down/down* 10 single count, *down/up* 10-second hold

LOOK OUT FOR: Placing your feet into too narrow or too wide of a V. Raising your heels up too high. (Keep them just an inch off the floor.) Not keeping your heels pressed together. Leaning too far forward as a result of bending your knees too much or not being aware of your posture. Rounding your shoulders and chest. Dropping your arms and not maintaining a T-shape. Sticking your butt out instead of keeping it in line with your heels.

NEED TO MODIFY? Tender knees or ankles: Don't bend your knees as much and reduce your range of movement *or* flatten your feet.

TRANSITION: Lower your feet and turn them in, fold your body over; and flow into exercise 6.

6. Ragdoll

Repeat exercise 4.

TRANSITION: Step your right foot and then your left foot back behind you; flow into exercise 7.

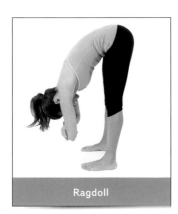

Ragdoll

7. Plank Bends

FOCUS: Core and shoulders

INTENTION: "I can do this. Stay calm and focus on the form."

GET IN POSITION: Begin in Plank position with your hands in line with your shoulders, palms flat and fingertips spread. Keep your feet and thighs together. Straighten your legs. Tip your heels forward, as if you are stretching your feet and your body is about to take off. Level your hips and keep your back flat. Tighten your abs by pulling your belly button in toward your spine. Tuck your hips slightly so your back feels protected. Keep your chest open, with your shoulders back and down, away from your ears. Your head should be in line with your spine. Focus on the floor. Your entire body should feel solid, as if you're stuck in a tube.

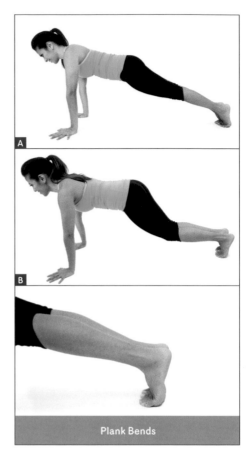

Plank Bends

GET MOVING: Continue to monitor the flatness of your body. Push away from the floor while maintaining good posture. Maintain straight legs. Maintaining a flat back, bend and stretch your knees and then straighten your legs. Make sure the bends are tiny as you keep the rest of your body solid. Keep your chest open and your head in line with your spine. Keep shifting your weight forward slightly.

SERIES: 5-second hold 20 single count, *bend/stretch* 5-second hold

LOOK OUT FOR: Keeping your hips too low or too high and arching or rounding your back as a result. Dropping your head. Rounding your shoulders. Placing your hands too close together or too far apart. Placing your hands too far forward and not in line with your shoulders. Bending your knees too much and sacrificing the flatness of your back. Being bouncy in your movements instead of controlled. Arching your back instead of engaging your abs and tucking your hips slightly. Forgetting to tip your heels forward.

NEED TO MODIFY? Tender wrists or tight shoulders: Do Forearm Plank (p. 66) instead. Tender back: Give yourself mini-breaks and be patient.

TRANSITION: Shift your weight and hips back and up; flow into exercise 8.

8. Down Dog

FOCUS: Hamstrings and back

BREATHING TECHNIQUE: Inhale your arms long and hips up/Exhale your shoulders down and heels toward the floor.

GET IN POSITION: Beginning in Plank position, make sure your hands are slightly in front of your shoulders. Your palms (parallel or slightly turned out) should be flat and your fingers spread. Keep your toes curled as you shift your weight back and lift your hips up toward the ceiling. As you start to lengthen your arms and legs, continue to press your palms and heels down. As your hips rise toward the ceiling, push the tops of your thighs back and stretch your heels down to the floor, lengthening your hamstrings. Straighten your knees but do not lock them. Maintain straight legs. (Soften your knees if your lower back or hamstrings are tight.) Rotate your elbows in to firm up the arms and shoulders. Maintain a long back. Keep your head in line with your arms; do not hang your head down. (Note: Imagine you're creating a teepee with your body!)

SERIES: 10-second hold

NEED TO MODIFY? Tender knees or tight back and hamstrings: Keep your legs bent and heels raised.

TRANSITION: Shift your weight forward and hands wider; flow into exercise 9.

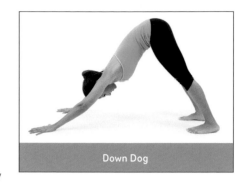

Down Dog

9. Push-Ups

FOCUS: Chest, arms, and core

INTENTION: "Even if it is tiny, it counts—and I'm getting stronger."

GET IN POSITION: Begin in Plank position with your hands wider than your shoulders, palms flat and fingertips spread. Keep your feet and thighs together. Straighten your legs. Tip your heels forward, as if you are stretching your feet and your body is about to take off. Level your hips and keep your

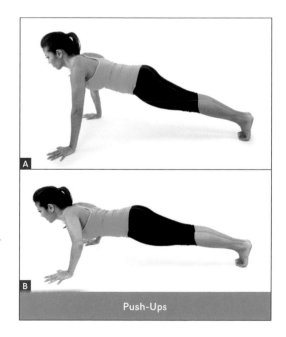

Push-Ups

back flat. Tighten your abs by pulling your belly button in toward your spine. Tuck your hips slightly so your back feels protected. Keep your chest open, with your shoulders back and down, away from your ears. Your head should be in line with your spine. Focus on the floor. Your entire body should feel solid, as if you're stuck in a tube.

GET MOVING: Bending your elbows and leading with your chest, lower your entire body to the floor and then straighten your arms to lift your entire body back up. Lower yourself as far as you can without sacrificing your form—even a mini push-up counts! Make sure you keep tipping your heels forward with every push-up. Maintain good posture and tap into your core strength for this workout.

SERIES: 20 single count, *down/up*

LOOK OUT FOR: Keeping your hips too low or too high and arching or rounding your back as a result. Dropping your head. Rounding your shoulders and not squeezing your shoulder blades together on the way down. Placing your hands too close together or too far apart. Placing your hands too far forward and not in line with your shoulders. Arching your back instead of engaging your abs and tucking your hips slightly. Forgetting to tip your heels forward. Giving up because you can manage only a tiny range of movement.

NEED TO MODIFY? Tender wrists or tight shoulders: Make fists and substitute them for your flat palms. Tender back: Give yourself mini-breaks and be patient *or* do Push-Up Bent Knees (p. 88) instead.

TRANSITION: Shift your weight back and hips up; flow into exercise 10.

10. Down Dog

Repeat exercise 8.

TRANSITION: Shift your weight forward and place your hands wider; flow into exercise 11.

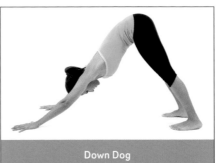
Down Dog

11. Tricep Push-up

FOCUS: Chest, arms, triceps, and core

INTENTION: "This is challenging, it's supposed to be, and I'm stepping up to it."

GET IN POSITION: Begin in Plank position with your hands in line with your shoulders, palms flat and fingertips spread. Keep your feet and thighs together. Straighten your legs. Tip your heels forward, as if you are stretching your feet and your body is about to take off. Level your hips and keep your back flat. Turn your fingertips out slightly. (Think two o'clock and ten o'clock.) Turn your elbows into your body to isolate your triceps. Tighten your abs by pulling your belly button in toward your spine. Tuck your hips slightly so your back feels protected. Keep your chest open, with your shoulders back and down, away from your ears. Your head should be in line with your spine. Focus on the floor. Your entire body should feel solid, as if you're stuck in a tube.

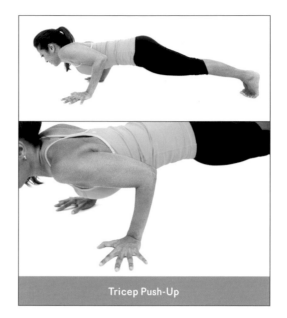

Tricep Push-Up

GET MOVING: Leading with your chest, bend your elbows down and in toward your body to lower your entire body to the floor and then straighten your arms to lift your entire body back up. Lower yourself as far as you can without sacrificing your form—even a mini push-up counts! Make sure you keep tipping your heels forward with every push-up. Maintain good posture and tap into your triceps and core strength for this workout. (This should feel different than your regular Push-Up as triceps are the focus.) Try to keep your body parallel to the floor.

SERIES: 20 single count, *down/up*

LOOK OUT FOR: Keeping your hips too low or too high and arching or rounding your back as a result. Dropping your head. Rounding your shoulders and not squeezing your shoulder blades together on the way down. Placing your hands too close together or too far apart. Placing your hands too far forward and not in line with your shoulders. Turning your elbows out instead of in toward your rib cage. Arching your back instead of engaging your abs and tucking your hips slightly. Forgetting to tip your heels forward. Giving up because you can manage only a tiny range of movement.

NEED TO MODIFY? Tender wrists or tight shoulders: Make fists and substitute them for your flat palms. Tender back: Give yourself mini-breaks and be patient *or* do Push-Up Bent Knees (p. 88) instead.

TRANSITION: Slowly lower your body and lie on your stomach; flow into exercise 12.

12. Cobra

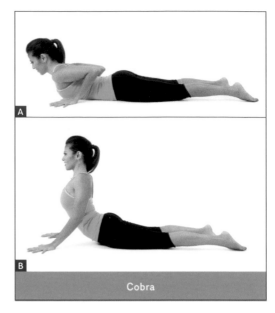

Cobra

FOCUS: Core and back

BREATHING TECHNIQUE: Inhale your chest up/Exhale your hips forward and shoulders back.

GET IN POSITION: Begin by lying on your stomach, propped on your forearms. Slide your hands back under your shoulders, keeping your palms flat and fingertips spread. Keep your elbows bent, hugging them tightly into your body. Keep your feet and knees hip-width apart. Press the tops of your feet, thighs, and hips firmly into the floor. Start to lengthen and straighten your arms while lifting your chest off the floor. Keep your shoulder blades back, puffing your ribs forward. Keep your hips connected to the floor and lift your upper body. (You might not be able to straighten your arms entirely, so feel free to keep your elbows slightly bent for comfort.) Firm up your butt and drive your hips forward while lifting your chest and stretching your abs. Twist your upper body to the right and to the left, lengthening your sides, and then return to center. (Repeat the movement twice.)

SERIES: 10-second hold

NEED TO MODIFY? Tender back: Do Cat/Cow (p. 99) instead.

TRANSITION: Shift your weight and rest back; flow into exercise 13.

13. Child's Pose

FOCUS: Shoulders and back

MANTRA: Love yourself dearly. Be yourself completely. Treat yourself occasionally.

BREATHING TECHNIQUE: Inhale and exhale; observe your chest rising and falling. Embrace a sense of calm.

GET IN POSITION: Begin by kneeling on the floor and sitting on your heels. Your feet should be comfortably together, with your knees apart and wider than your hips. Fold your upper body

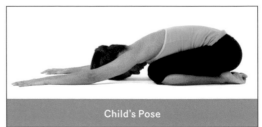

Child's Pose

forward between your thighs and bring your forehead to the floor. Reach your straight arms forward with your palms down. Release your shoulders toward the floor.

SERIES: 10-second hold

NEED TO MODIFY? Tender knees: Place a pillow under your hamstrings for elevation *or* play around with the placement of your knees until you feel comfortable.

TRANSITION: Bring your arms forward to help you turn and lie on your right side; flow into exercise 14.

14. L-Shape (Left)

FOCUS: Glutes and hips

INTENTION: "How fun: I'm lying down and still getting a great workout."

GET IN POSITION: Begin by lying on your right side. Bend your right elbow and lift your forearm so that you can rest your head on your hand. Adjust your elbow and hand placement to be comfortably in line with your shoulder. Stack your feet and knees and bend your knees at a 90-degree angle. Bring your knees up toward your chest, lining them up just shy of your hips (an inch away from being right in front of your hips). Play around with the angle if you need to and get comfortable. Lean forward and press your left hand into the floor. Tighten your abs by pulling your belly button in toward your spine. Your body should feel solid and grounded. Angle your shin up. (Keep your knee down and tilt your left shin and foot up toward the ceiling.) Point or flex your left foot. (Your choice for comfort, but don't leave it loose/hanging.) Focus forward.

GET MOVING: Lean forward into your left hand and activate your abs. Lift and lower your leg, maintaining the angled shape. Keep your left foot higher than your knee with your knee angled down. The key is to find your ideal range. (Slightly higher than your hip, but not too high! And not too low; don't touch your bottom knee!)

SERIES: 20 double count, *up/up/down/ down* 20 single count, *up/down* 20

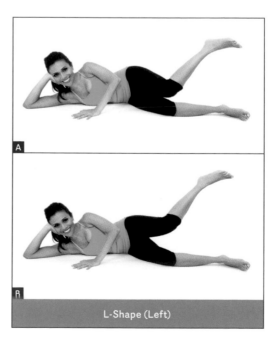

L-Shape (Left)

pulses, *up/up* 10 multi-count, *up/up/up/down* 10 single count, *up/down* 10 pulses, *up/up* 10-second hold

LOOK OUT FOR: Lifting your left leg too high. Forgetting to keep your shin angled up. Dropping your foot instead of keeping it above your knee. Swinging your leg instead of making precise movements. Rushing and skipping the strategic tempo.

NEED TO MODIFY? Tender back: Do All Fours (p. 61) instead.

TRANSITION: Sit up and extend your legs; flow into exercise 15.

15. Seated Twist (Left)

FOCUS: Glutes and hips

BREATHING TECHNIQUE: Inhale your knee to the right/ Exhale your left hip back.

GET IN POSITION: Begin by sitting on the floor with your spine perpendicular to your legs. Your right leg should be extended in front of you with your right foot flexed and your toes pointing up to the ceiling. Cross your left leg over your right. Bend your left knee and use your hands to help you place your left foot flat on the floor next to your right knee. Facing forward, with your right arm, hug your bent knee in toward your chest. Press your left hand into the floor (next to your left hip) and pull your left hip back. Keep hugging in your knee as you twist your left knee toward your right shoulder. The twist is like a push/pull between your knee pulling up to the right and your left hip pushing down toward the floor and back to the left. Both arms should assist with lengthening. Keep your spine straight. Tighten your abs by pulling your belly button in toward your spine. Lift your abs and chest up and away from your hips. Keep your chest open, with your shoulders back and down, away from your ears. Keep your head in line with your spine. Focus forward.

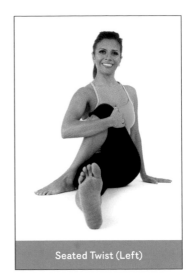

Seated Twist (Left)

SERIES: 10-second hold

NEED TO MODIFY? Tender knees or tight back: Skip crossing your left leg over your right. Just keep your legs parallel as you bend your left knee and draw your left heel back to your left hip.

TRANSITION: Lie down; flow into exercise 16.

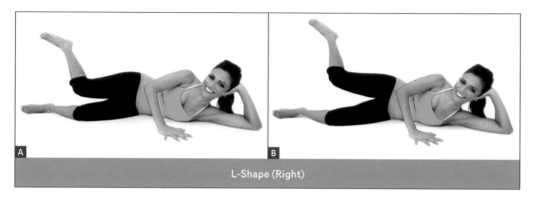

L-Shape (Right)

16. L-Shape (Right)

Repeat exercise 14, this time lying on your left side and lifting your right leg.

TRANSITION: Sit up and extend your legs; flow into exercise 17.

17. Seated Twist (Right)

Repeat exercise 15, extending your left leg and bending your right knee.

TRANSITION: Slide your right foot over; flow into exercise 18.

18. Seated Triangle (Right/Left)

FOCUS: Glutes and hips

BREATHING TECHNIQUE: Inhale as you reach your arms to the left/Exhale as you pull your right hip back and down. Inhale as you reach your arms to the right/Exhale as you pull your left hip back and down.

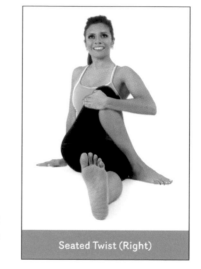

Seated Twist (Right)

GET IN POSITION: Begin in a cross-legged seated position. Using your hands, gently place your right ankle on top of your left knee, aligning your right shin with your left shin. Flex your right foot. Adjust your left foot so that it is in line with your right knee. (This creates a "triangle" between your thighs.) Don't worry if there is a lot of space between your right knee and your left foot and you don't "look" flexible; the feet and knees being aligned is more important. Place your palms down on the floor by your sides. Use your hands to help you push your hips back as you fold your upper body forward. Draw your chest toward your shins. Walk both of your arms to your left side, in line with your right foot. Continue to reach and walk your fingertips and arms out to the left as you resist and press your right hip down toward the floor. Repeat the movement on your left side.

SERIES: 10-second hold, right side (right leg on top, arms to your left) 10-second hold, right side (left leg on top, arms to your right)

NEED TO MODIFY? Tight hips: Do Lying T-Stretch (p. 60) instead.

TRANSITION: Lie flat on your back and extend your legs up to the ceiling; flow into exercise 19.

19. Frog

FOCUS: Inner thighs

INTENTION: "Go, me! I'm lying here targeting that forgotten spot on the body. Feels great!"

GET IN POSITION: Begin by lying flat on your back with your legs straight and perpendicular to the ceiling. Your arms should be resting by your sides. Place your feet in a V-shape, with your heels together and your toes apart. Keep your heels together as you bend your knees and lower your feet toward your butt. Spread your knees and thighs as wide as possible. (Think Plié.) Keep your heels together and in line with your tailbone.

GET MOVING: Bend your knees and lower your feet toward your butt and back up to your original position. Keep your heels together! Imagine your heels are drawing a straight line up and down a wall. Continue to press your knees and thighs apart. (How far your knees can spread will depend on your hip flexibility.) Keep your back flat.

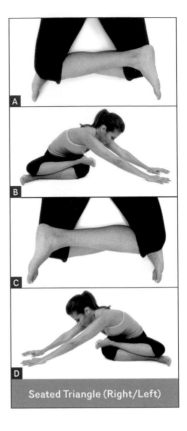

Seated Triangle (Right/Left)

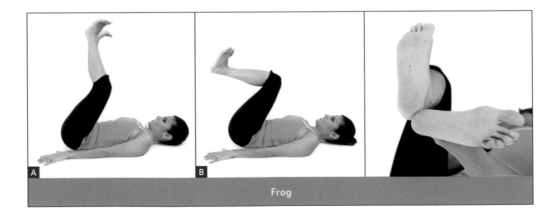

Frog

SERIES: 10 double count, *down/down/up/up* 10 single count, *down/up* 10 pulses, *up/up* 10 double count, i*n/in/out/out* (Keep your heels together as you bring your knees and thighs together and then apart.) 10 single count, *in/out* (Keep your heels together as you bring your knees and thighs together and then apart.) 10 pulses, *out/out* (Keep your heels together and thighs apart and press your knees and thighs out and away from you—tiny movements, an inch in range.) 10 single count, *up/down*, full range 5-second hold (Bring your feet down as low as possible; press your knees out wide one last time.)

LOOK OUT FOR: Separating your heels. Dropping just your feet instead of opening and bending your knees wide enough that your feet naturally come down. Arching your back and not engaging and grounding your core.

NEED TO MODIFY? Tender hips: Do Seated Leg Lifts (p. 91) instead.

TRANSITION: Stay flat on your back and bend your knees; flow into exercise 20.

20. Happy Baby

FOCUS: Inner thighs

BREATHING TECHNIQUE: Inhale and push your feet into your hands/Exhale and pull your knees down.

GET IN POSITION: Begin by lying flat on your back, hugging your knees into your chest comfortably. (How much space is between your knees depends on your flexibility and comfort.) Lift your feet up and back toward your shoulders, drawing your knees even closer to your chest. Using your hands, grab the outer edges of your feet. Flex your feet and let your inner thighs spread apart even more. Keep your knees wider than your torso and bring them up toward your shoulders. Keep your ankles in line with your knees and your shins perpendicular to the floor. Keep your back flat on the floor. Create resistance by pushing your feet into your hands while pulling your knees and legs down. Rock from side to side.

SERIES: 10-second hold

NEED TO MODIFY? Hard time holding onto your feet: Hold onto the insides of your shins or thighs instead.

TRANSITION: Lower your legs and feet flat onto the floor; flow into exercise 21.

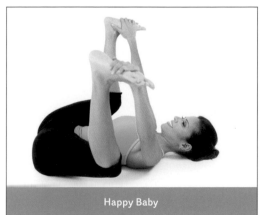

Happy Baby

21. Lying Diamond Stretch

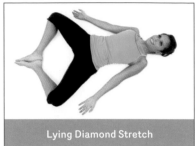

Lying Diamond Stretch

FOCUS: Hips

BREATHING TECHNIQUE: Inhale—your chest rises and your feet slide in/Exhale to let your knees drop and settle back down.

GET IN POSITION: Begin by lying flat on your back. Bend your knees and draw your feet toward your butt, keeping your feet flat on the floor. Create a diamond shape with your legs by separating your knees and placing the soles of your feet together in front of your groin. Move your feet closer in or farther away from you to find your "sweet spot." Let your knees fall toward the floor. Keep your arms straight alongside your torso with your palms up. Avoid pressing your knees down with your hands.

SERIES: 10-second hold

NEED TO MODIFY? Tight hips: Elevate your knees with pillows.

TRANSITION: Bring your knees together and lift your legs; flow into exercise 22.

22. Lower Ab Series

FOCUS: Core

INTENTION: "I am grounded and able to pace myself and successfully make it through this challenge."

GET IN POSITION: Begin by lying flat on your back with your legs straight and perpendicular to the ceiling. Keep your legs pressed together and bend both of your knees at a 90-degree angle. Keep your knees in line with your hips and your feet across from your knees. Flex your feet and keep your feet and knees pressed firmly together. With your arms by your sides, use your hands to grab the edges of your mat. (If you don't have a mat, ground your arms by flattening your palms or wrists into the floor.) (Note: It should feel as if you are trying to pull the mat down and out from underneath you, but your flat back is stopping it from happening!) Press your lower back into the floor. Keep your head in line with your spine. Focus up. (Note: Move through the series swiftly; don't take too long of a break between sets!)

GET MOVING: Using your hands to help you press your back down and tap into your core strength, start to lower your legs and then raise them back up. Maintain a grounded back. (That is your #1 priority!) Keep all movements controlled and isolate your abs. (By keeping your back flat, you may manage only a small range of motion.) When moving, it should feel as if you are testing the edge of your strength. (Lower your legs as far as you can without arching your back.) Your abs workout will fall into place nicely if your lower back feels safe and protected. Keep creating resistance with your hands on the floor to help you maintain a flat back. During the holds, make sure to check in, grounding your back and perfecting your form.

SERIES: Set 1: *Bent Leg Down/Up* Maintaining a 90-degree angle in your knees, lower and lift your legs. 5-second hold (Make sure your form is correct and your back feels secure.) 10 double count, *down/down/up/up* 10 single count, *down/up* Rest (a couple of seconds; not too long!) Set 2: *Bent Leg Out/In* Begin in a 90-degree angle and then push your knees and legs away from you and pull them back in. (If your back and core strength allow it, extend your legs completely straight and challenge yourself with a full range.) 5-second hold (Make sure your form is correct and your back feels secure) 10 double count, *out/out/in/in* 10 single count, *out/in* Rest (a couple of seconds; not too long!) Set 3: *Bent Leg Down/Up/Out/In* Begin in a 90-degree angle and move your legs *down/up* and then push your legs *out/in*. (Think of it as a combination of the first two sets.) Make sure the 90-degree angle is your foundation point every time! 5-second hold (Make sure your form is correct and your back feels secure.) 10 single count, *down/up/out/in* Rest (a couple of seconds; not too long!)

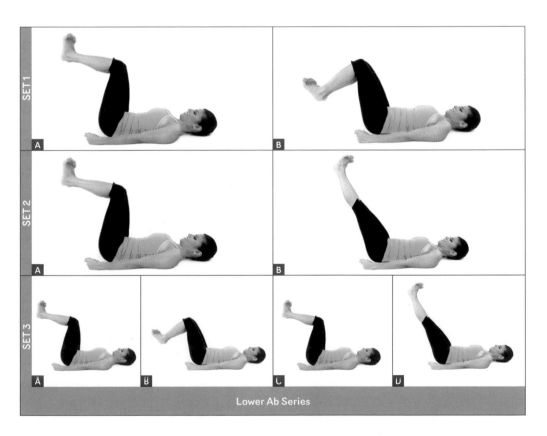

Lower Ab Series

Set 4: *Straight Leg Hold* Extend your legs away from your hips, keeping your legs straight. Place your feet in a V-shape, with your heels together and your toes apart. Lower your legs—only go as low as feels safe for your back! 20-second hold Set 5: *Lower Abs Jumps* Raise your legs straight toward the ceiling, perpendicular to your spine, and point your toes. Keep your legs together and bend your knees slightly. Lift your hips and lower back off the floor and then lower them while maintaining straight legs (with a microbend in the knees), toes in line with your hips. (Note: It should feel as if your butt jumps off the floor and you are hitting the same spot on the ceiling with your toes every time.) 10 single count, *up/down* 10 pulses, *up/up* 5-second hold (hips up off the floor!) Rest (a couple of seconds; not too long!) Set 6: *Abs Rolls* Bend your knees and draw them in toward your chest and drop your feet toward your butt. Roll your knees and hips up to your chest and then back down toward the floor. 10 double count, *in/in/down/down* 10 single count, *in/down* 5-second hold (hips up off of floor!) Rest (a couple of seconds; not too long!)

LOOK OUT FOR: Sets 1–4: Arching your back and not grounding your back into the floor. Worrying about how low your legs are going and lowering them too much. Not using

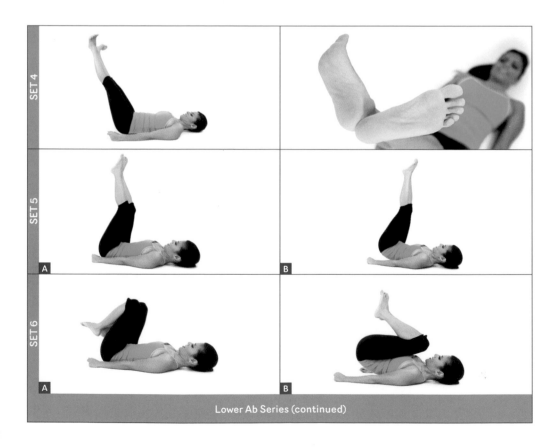

Lower Ab Series (continued)

your arms and hands to help keep your back in position. **Sets 5–6:** Swinging your legs instead of making deliberate, controlled movements. Not using your arms and hands to help create resistance.

NEED TO MODIFY? Tender back: Reduce your range and/or bring your feet closer to your butt *or* just keep your back pressed into the floor, and hold for 1-minute intervals *or* just do sets 5 and 6.

TRANSITION: Lower your legs; flow into exercise 23.

23. Spinal Twist (Right/Left)

FOCUS: Core and back

BREATHING TECHNIQUE: Inhale your right knee down/Exhale your right hip back and right arm down. Inhale your left knee down/Exhale your left hip back and left arm down.

GET IN POSITION: Begin by lying flat on your back with your legs straight and your feet hip-width apart. Stretch your arms out across from your shoulders, forming a T-shape, with your palms facing down. Bend your right knee in toward your chest. Use your left hand to pull your right knee toward your left side and down toward the floor. Keep your chest open and your right arm steady in its original position. Keep your hips squared and avoid aggressively pushing your knee down. Keep your toes pointed. Enjoy a natural twist in your back. Repeat the movement with your left leg.

SERIES: 10-second hold, right side (twisting your right knee to the left) 10-second hold, left side (twisting your left knee to the right)

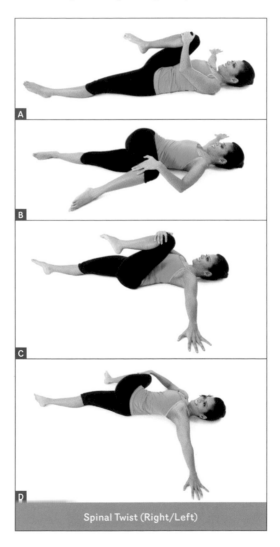

Spinal Twist (Right/Left)

NEED TO MODIFY? Tender back: Lower bent knees together to the right and left instead of keeping one leg straight.

TRANSITION: Turn back to center; flow into exercise 24.

24. Savasana

FOCUS: Total body awareness and relaxation

MANTRA: Love yourself dearly. Be yourself completely. Treat yourself occasionally.

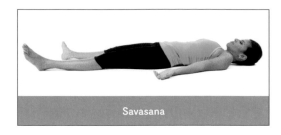
Savasana

BREATHING TECHNIQUE: Inhale and tense up your body: tighten your legs and arms and clench your fists and face/Exhale and relax all your muscles at once. Embrace the sense of peace.

GET IN POSITION: Begin by lying flat on your back with your legs straight and feet spread comfortably apart. Rest your arms comfortably by your sides, palms up. Feel your chest and heart open and keep your eyes closed.

SERIES: 10 breaths, *inhale/exhale* Make sure to take full, long breaths. Once you're done, bend your knees and turn onto your side, slowly making your way up.

NEED TO MODIFY? Hopefully, you don't! Just be patient and rest, allow yourself this time, and don't rush it!

THE POST-WORKOUT

1 **Post-Workout Recap:**

Be proud of yourself. It's easy to take being chill for granted. Instead, you took the time to recognize it and be present for a fulfilling workout.

Did my emotional weight change?

☐ YES   ☐ NO

Did I accomplish my workout intention?

☐ YES   ☐ NO

Is there a change in my physical body?

☐ YES   ☐ NO

2 **My Post-Workout Mood Is:**

(Write down, think, or say out loud.)

_____

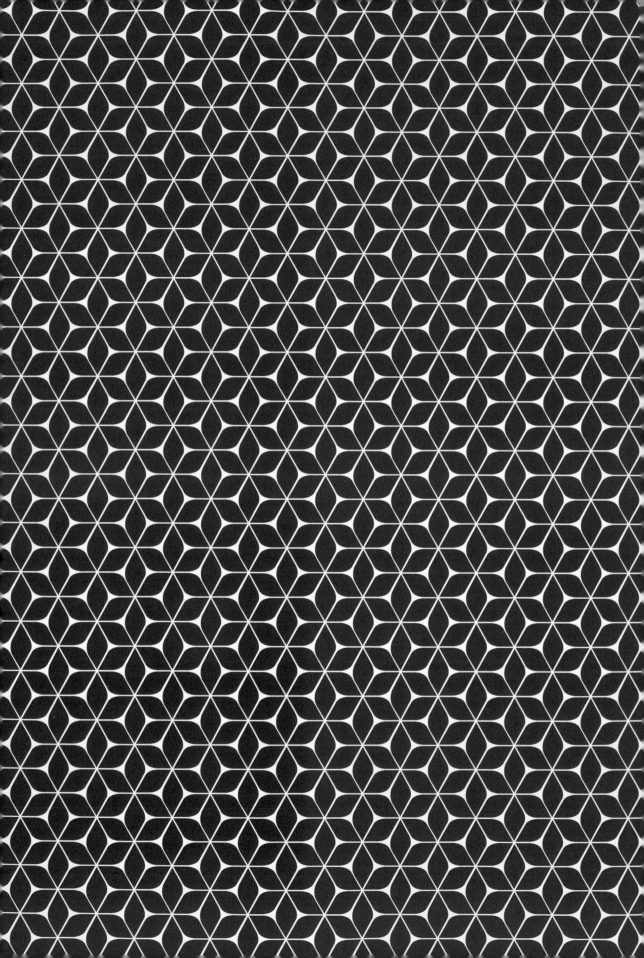

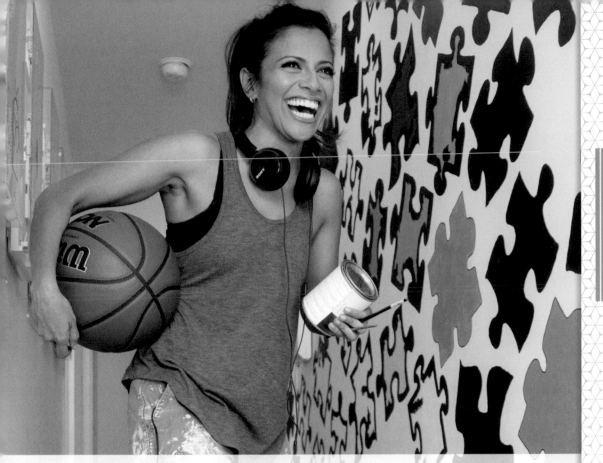

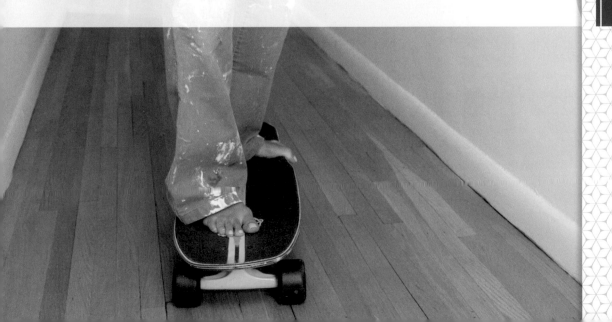

— CHAPTER 7 —

THE HAPPINESS WORKOUT

HAPPINESS

THE HAPPINESS EXERCISES

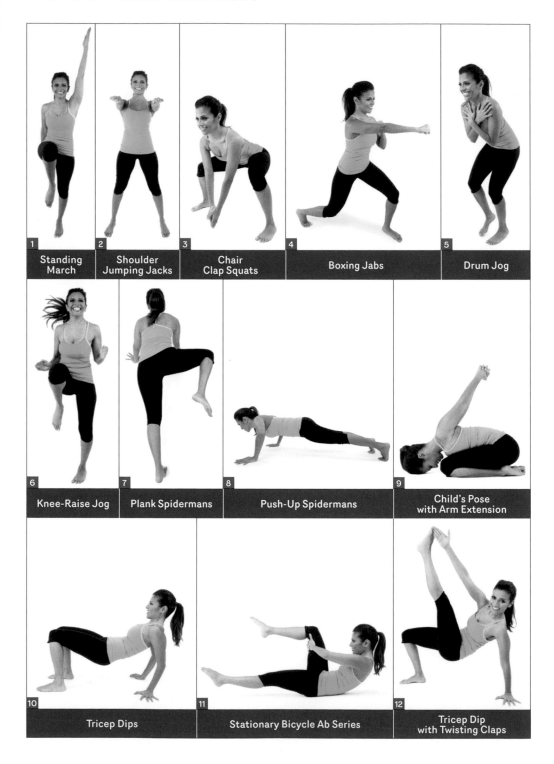

1. Standing March
2. Shoulder Jumping Jacks
3. Chair Clap Squats
4. Boxing Jabs
5. Drum Jog
6. Knee-Raise Jog
7. Plank Spidermans
8. Push-Up Spidermans
9. Child's Pose with Arm Extension
10. Tricep Dips
11. Stationary Bicycle Ab Series
12. Tricep Dip with Twisting Claps

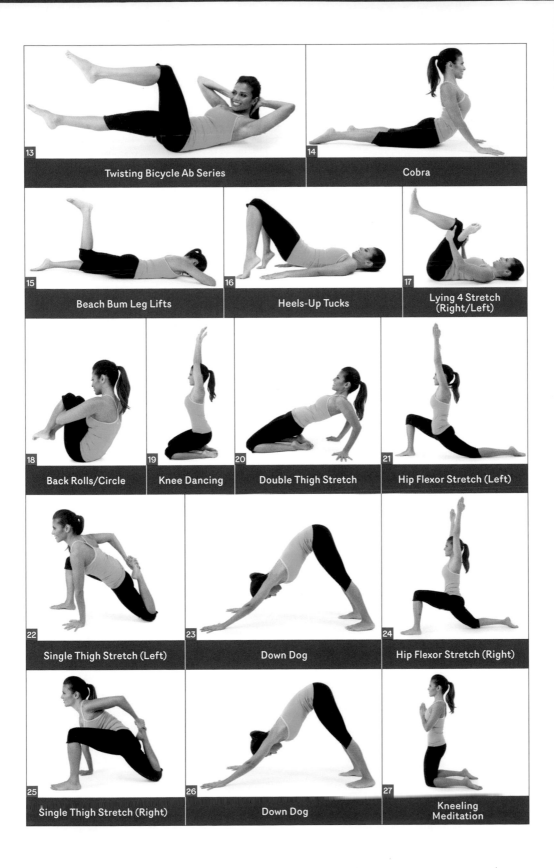

13 Twisting Bicycle Ab Series

14 Cobra

15 Beach Bum Leg Lifts

16 Heels-Up Tucks

17 Lying 4 Stretch (Right/Left)

18 Back Rolls/Circle

19 Knee Dancing

20 Double Thigh Stretch

21 Hip Flexor Stretch (Left)

22 Single Thigh Stretch (Left)

23 Down Dog

24 Hip Flexor Stretch (Right)

25 Single Thigh Stretch (Right)

26 Down Dog

27 Kneeling Meditation

Happiness is an emotion that reminds me of helium in a balloon—it can automatically lift you up into the sky. Your emotional weight should be just as light!

Happiness is all about pleasure and feeling elated. Perhaps you accomplished a long-term goal you've worked incredibly hard for, and are savoring the thrill of a job well done. Perhaps you've just fallen in love with the best person ever. Perhaps a friend got unexpected good news, and you're ecstatic that you can share the moment. What is the thing and/or person creating this joy in your life? That is what I want you to reflect on.

What is the emotional weight of that thought and its resulting mood, and how is it manifesting in your physical body?

THE PRE-WORKOUT

1 **I Am Feeling:**

- ☐ Blessed
- ☐ Blissful
- ☐ Breezy
- ☐ Charmed
- ☐ Cheerful
- ☐ Content
- ☐ Delighted
- ☐ Ebullient
- ☐ Ecstatic
- ☐ Effervescent
- ☐ Elated
- ☐ Enchanted
- ☐ Enraptured
- ☐ Enthralled

- ☐ Euphoric
- ☐ Excited
- ☐ Exhilarated
- ☐ Festive
- ☐ Glad
- ☐ Gleeful
- ☐ Gratified
- ☐ Happy
- ☐ Inspired
- ☐ Jaunty
- ☐ Jolly
- ☐ Joyful
- ☐ Jubilation
- ☐ Lighthearted

- ☐ Merry
- ☐ Pleased
- ☐ Radiant
- ☐ Rejoicing
- ☐ Rhapsodic
- ☐ Satisfied
- ☐ Smiley
- ☐ Spirited
- ☐ Sunshiny
- ☐ Thrilled
- ☐ Tickled
- ☐ Transported

2 **My Current Mood Is:**

_____

3 **My Emotional Weight Is:**

1	5	10
Light	Neutral	Heavy

4 **My Physical Symptoms Are:**

- ☐ Bounciness
- ☐ Clarity
- ☐ Confident Movement
- ☐ Easy Breathing
- ☐ Easy Digestion
- ☐ Endorphin Release

- ☐ Evenness
- ☐ Flushing
- ☐ Glowing
- ☐ Increased Dopamine
- ☐ Increased Energy
- ☐ Muscle Relaxation
- ☐ Need to Move

- ☐ Sense of Well-Being
- ☐ Smiling
- ☐ Sparkling
- ☐ Steadiness
- ☐ Tingling
- ☐ Touchy-Feely

TEN COMMON HAPPINESS THOUGHTS

- I am so full of happiness that I could just burst! I want everybody in the world to be as happy as I am!
- Have you ever seen a baby with such yummy, pinchable cheeks? Just looking at that darling little face fills me with joy.
- My daughter worked so hard to learn Mandarin. When I heard her confidently talking to a Chinese friend, I nearly burst into tears! I was so proud.
- I can't believe you're finally home for good!
- Nothing tastes better than a really good piece of chocolate after I just spent an hour in the gym.
- School's out for the summer!
- I got the job of my dreams. I can't believe it. I did well!
- I am so lucky. I can't believe I got it!
- I won! I actually won! I mean, did you hear me? I can repeat the story all day—I won!
- I love you, I love you, I love you!

THE WORKOUT

1 Mantra For Happiness:

Thank you.

Being happy is just the best! What I love about being happy is everyone's jokes are funnier, everybody seems nicer, and all seems well with the world. Even my body seems to be in optimal shape. When I'm happy, my cheer spreads internally and externally. It's contagious in the best possible way.

Usually, what gives birth to my happy mood is something or someone special to me. However big or small—a subway coming on time, a generous compliment from a client, getting the apartment of my dreams, a friend helping me put together my Ikea furniture—it is deserving of acknowledgment and gratitude. Sometimes life is complicated, so a simple happy moment that springs up and makes you feel like the sun is shining directly on you is always something to be grateful for.

Our culture loves to say "Thank you." From Hallmark cards to 1-800-Flowers, we have companies built on the premise that favorable thoughts and expressions of gratitude are heartfelt and good. We are quick to say "Thank you" to the waitress, the cashier, the teacher, the president, and God. But sometimes the people closest to us, who give us a foundation for happiness and pleasure in our lives, get forgotten, lost in the mix, or taken for granted.

To be fair, we do thank our friends and family lovingly around birthdays, anniversaries, and holidays. But the phrase "Thank you" seems different somehow when we acknowledge the people closest to us. I have to admit I was astonished when I looked at the *New Oxford American Dictionary*'s second definition of the word *thank*. The first definition is "to express gratitude to (someone)," and the second is "used ironically to assign blame or responsibility for something."

But then I realized that, within the context of our culture, this notion does make sense. When it comes to our sometimes fast and impatient society, we tend to assign blame or responsibility for our life's failures to our closest loved ones. But our successes? Oh . . . *we* take full credit for those.

My parents always say, "The only thing constant in life is change and death." Talking so freely about the unreliability of things and people I loved, as well as the inevitability of death, led to conversations that often seemed cold, hopeless, scary, and even taboo. But now, I can truly understand the cycle of life and death and the importance of thanking people. There are many people I love, and one day they will be gone. I want to recognize this cycle and appreciate these people, whether they are strangers or family, for what they have given me.

Take my parents. I thanked them all the time as a little girl, looking at them with big, admiring eyes. I didn't thank them much as a rebellious teenager in high school. I did thank them when they supported me in college, but I didn't thank them when they didn't fully agree with my career choices. I do thank them now. I thanked my best friend from childhood when I was a hormonal teenager who needed to vent. But she didn't get thanked during my career-focused twenties. Now she's getting thanked in full for being there by my side during hard times in my thirties. When I put the "Thank you" mantra into play is when I feel most suffused with that heavenly feeling that all is right with the world. This is because it allows me to share my happiness with those who mean the most to me.

Thanking and appreciating people, especially those closest to us, comes in cycles. The emotions and realities we associate with them are not constants; they will change in conjunction with our lives. To understand this is to embrace my parents' words of wisdom: "The only thing constant in life is change and death."

Which is why the "Thank you" mantra is so important. Our parents were once children like us, and someday we may be (or may already be) parents ourselves. We may someday be in our friend's shoes. Our parents and friends will die and so will we. So welcome this cycle, and because words do matter, make an active effort to thank your family and friends—not just when you're happy. Whenever you want to! Nothing makes people happier than to be acknowledged, whether it's because they brought you chicken soup when you had the flu, or because you know they'll listen to you vent when your boss is being a pill, or even just *because*!

I don't always understand or agree with my family and friends, but no matter what, they are a part of my life. When you're feeling happy, take the time to acknowledge how lucky you are to be in that ebullient, singing-in-the-rain kind of state, and then express your gratitude to that person (or people!) who make a difference in your life.

2 How to Use the Mantra

Since this mantra is all about gratitude, what I'd like you to do is say "Thank you" to your own body. When's the last time you looked at your skin or your muscles or your hair with appreciation and marveled at how you look? So often, we take our bodies for granted until something goes wrong. Or we constantly criticize its faults, and then get frustrated when things aren't working properly. Thanking your own body for giving you the strength and support you need to complete this workout will not only heighten your happiness; it will encourage you to treat it as well as you know it should be treated.

Repeat the "Thank you" mantra as you recognize your body, and apply your ebullient state of mind to a joy-filled workout. Use your endorphins and increased dopamine levels as fuel to capitalize on your happiness.

3 Why the Happiness Workout

By now you have taken the time to reflect on the source of your happiness and how it is making you shine emotionally and physically.

Happiness makes people feel light and buoyant, so use this workout to heighten your happiness. Feel as if you are the world's most joyous balloon, rising up to the heavens and turning your head to the sun on a lovely spring day.

The flow of this series is designed for you to tap into the fun of your supremely positive mood. Enjoy every minute of it!

Embrace your mood, repeat the mantra, and let it provide you with the happiness to focus in on this breezy and cheer-enhancing routine.

4 My Happiness Workout Intention (Emotional or Physical) Is:
(Write down, think, or say out loud.)

_____

MUSIC

Choose music that will help you enjoy that extra kick in your step and your happiness even more. Here are a few suggestions that you'll love to sing along to:

1960s: "Brown-Eyed Girl" ▪ Van Morrison

1970s: "Hot Stuff" ▪ Donna Summer

1980s: "Love Shack" ▪ B-52's

1990s: "Groove Is In The Heart" ▪ Deee-Lite

2000s: "I Gotta Feeling" ▪ Black Eyed Peas

2010s: "Happy" ▪ Pharrell

5 The Happiness Exercises

1. Standing March

FOCUS: Warm-up, total body cardio, and awareness

INTENTION: "I'm going to have fun marching to my own beat."

GET IN POSITION: Begin by standing with your feet hip-width apart. Keep your feet parallel, with your toes in front of your heels. Maintain straight legs. Point your tailbone down. Tighten your abs by pulling your belly button in toward your spine. Stand tall as you lengthen your abs and chest up and

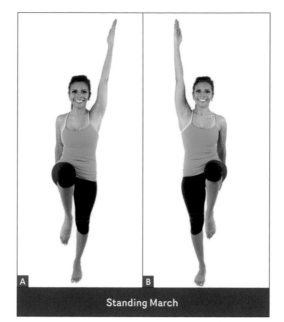

Standing March

away from your hips. Keep your chest open, with your shoulders back and down, away from your ears. Your arms should be straight down by your sides, palms facing in toward your body. Keep your head in line with your spine. Focus forward.

GET MOVING: Start marching by lifting your right knee and your left arm up to the ceiling. Then, switch sides, lifting your left knee and your right arm up to the ceiling. Keep your legs parallel as your knees alternate and come into your chest. Bring your knees up higher than your hips and keep your toes pointed. Keep your arms straight and parallel as they alternate and reach up to the ceiling. Bring your arms up above your head and keep your palms facing in toward your body. Move with precision—act as if you have to stay in the same exact spot every time you move. Engage your core and increase your tempo.

SERIES: 1-minute march (As many steps in form as you can.)

LOOK OUT FOR: Moving too slowly. (The idea is to get the heart rate up!) Not keeping your legs and arms parallel. Lifting your legs with your hip flexors instead of tapping into your core strength.

NEED TO MODIFY? Tender knees or back: Reduce your marching range and don't lift your knees as high.

TRANSITION: Jump into exercise 2.

2. Shoulder Jumping Jacks

FOCUS: Total body cardio

INTENTION: "My mood is even giving my normal jumping jacks an upgrade!"

GET IN POSITION: Begin by standing with your feet wider than your hips. Keep your feet parallel, with your toes in front of your heels. Point your tailbone down. Tighten your abs by pulling your belly button in toward your spine. Stand tall as you lengthen your abs and chest up and away from your hips. Keep your chest open, with your shoulders back and down, away from your ears. Raise your arms straight up across from your shoulders in a T-shape with your palms facing down. Keep your head in line with your spine. Focus forward.

GET MOVING: Jump your feet in, bringing your arms in front of you. Jump your feet out wider than your hips, lifting your arms out to a T-shape. Continue jumping your feet wider than your hips with your arms out and then your feet back together and arms forward. Keep in mind that whenever your feet are together, your arms are in front of you. Jump high, wide, and fast. (Note: This is hard to coordinate at first; just practice.)

SERIES: 20 single count, *out/in*

LOOK OUT FOR: Moving too slowly. (The idea is to get the heart rate up!) Not jumping your feet wide enough. Being sloppy with your posture. (Jump with confidence!) Getting frustrated with your coordination.

NEED TO MODIFY? Tender knees or back: Do Standing March (p. 169) instead.

TRANSITION: Keep your legs together on the last jump and squat down; flow into exercise 3.

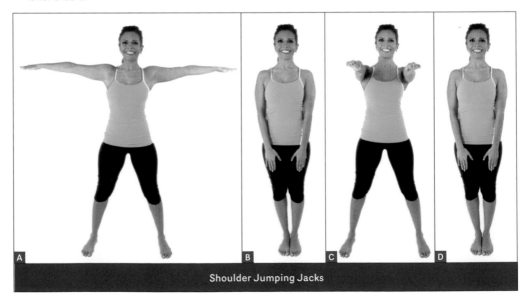

Shoulder Jumping Jacks

3. Chair Clap Squats

FOCUS: Total body cardio, thighs, and glutes

INTENTION: "This is hard and fun; I'm in the zone."

GET IN POSITION: Begin by standing in Chair Pose with your feet and knees together. Keep your feet parallel, with your toes in front of your heels. Keep your knees in line with your heels as you bend your knees and drop your hips, trying to get your thighs parallel to the floor. Press your feet firmly into

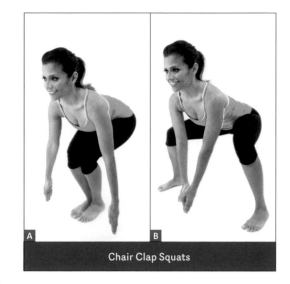

Chair Clap Squats

the floor. Lean forward slightly with your upper body until your back and thighs form a 90-degree angle. Keep your back flat and reach your straight arms down toward the floor. Tighten your abs by pulling your belly button in toward your spine. Your arms should be parallel to your shoulders, with your shoulders back and down, away from your ears. Face your palms toward one another and reach through your fingertips. Keep your tailbone down. Put more pressure on your heels, shifting your weight back. Your head should be in line with your spine. Focus forward.

GET MOVING: Jump your bent legs out to the sides into a wide squat (think wide-legged chair pose) as you bring your arms and palms together between your legs, continuing to reach toward the floor with your palms in. Jump back and forth between a wide-legged chair pose with your arms and palms together and a regular chair pose with your arms apart on either side of your body. Throughout the movement, maintain chair pose angles in your body. Keep your abs engaged and your core steady. Try to stay at the same height/angle with each jump out/in. Make sure your toes stay in line with the direction of your knees. (A good trick is to only pay attention to the coordination of your arms, or you can get thrown off! Think "hands together, hands apart" and your leg jump will become natural.)

SERIES: 20 single count, *out/in* (Jump out and in.)

LOOK OUT FOR: Being too bouncy and not tapping into the steadiness and strength of your jump. Leaning forward and sticking your butt out. Bad posture. Jumping unevenly. (Put the same effort into each leg.) Turning your feet out instead of keeping them parallel.

NEED TO MODIFY? Tender knees: Stay up higher *or* skip jumping and step out and in instead.

TRANSITION: Keep your legs wide on the last jump (wide chair pose); flow into exercise 4.

4. Boxing Jabs

FOCUS: Total body cardio and arms

INTENTION: "I have power and stamina."

GET IN POSITION: Begin in Plié. Keep both of your feet out at a 45-degree angle. (Think two o'clock and ten o'clock.) Bend your knees and drop your hips. Try to lower your hips so that they are in line with your knees. Press your feet firmly into the floor, toes in front of your heels. Lean forward slightly with your upper body. Tighten your abs by pulling your belly button in toward your spine. Keep your back flat. Keep your chest open, with your shoulders back and down, away from your ears. Bend your arms at a 90-degree angle and clench your fists. Angle your arms toward one another (kind of like a sumo wrestler's stance). Your head should be in line with your spine. Focus forward.

GET MOVING: Twist your upper and lower body to the left as you rotate your right hip to the left and raise onto the ball of your right foot. (It's as if you are twisting and turning into a lunge.) Jab your right arm across your body to the left. Keep your right arm at shoulder height. Get your hips and abs involved in the twist. Maintain a low squat position. Make sure your toes stay in line with the direction of your knees. Maintain your posture and tap into your core strength. Try to stay at the same height/angle with each jab as you twist from side to side.

SERIES: 20 single count jabs *right/left*

LOOK OUT FOR: Not jabbing with strength and power. (Imagine knocking someone out or breaking through a wall!) Bad posture. Jabbing unevenly. (Put the same effort into

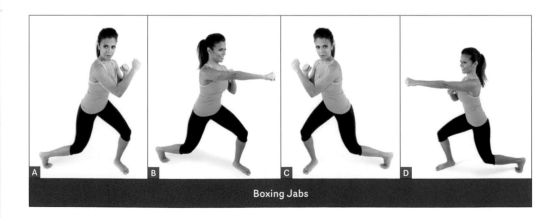

Boxing Jabs

each jab.) Forgetting about your non-jabbing arm staying tight and ready. Feeling loose in your body instead of feeling grounded.

NEED TO MODIFY? Tender shoulders: Don't extend your arms as far. Tender knees: Stay up higher.

TRANSITION: Stand up with your legs together; flow into exercise 5.

5. Drum Jog

FOCUS: Total body cardio

INTENTION: "I'm drumming up my mood, celebrating my internal music."

GET IN POSITION: Begin by standing with your feet hip-width apart. Keep your feet parallel, with your toes in front of your heels. Raise your heels slightly. Bend your knees and drop your hips. (Your body should be at the same level as in chair pose.) Lean your upper body forward slightly until your back and thighs form a 90-degree angle. Tighten your abs by pulling your belly button in toward your spine. Cross your arms across your chest, making the letter *X*. Keep your chest open, with your shoulders back and down, away from your ears. Keep your head in line with your spine. Focus forward.

GET MOVING: Start jogging really fast—imagine your feet are drumsticks and you are beating the floor with your feet. The goal is to go super-fast, alternating right and left. (Think a mini quick step—a fast jog.) Arms stay hugged in tight across your chest. Throughout the movement, maintain the chair pose angle in your body. Make sure your toes stay in line with direction of your knees. Move with precision—act as if you have to stay in same exact spot every time you move. Engage your core and increase your tempo.

SERIES: 30-second jog (As many quick steps in form as you can.)

LOOK OUT FOR: Moving too slowly. (The idea is to keep the heart rate up!) Not staying steady and maintaining tight rhythm.

NEED TO MODIFY? Tender knees or back: Do Standing March (p. 169) instead.

TRANSITION: Stay standing and quickly switch focus; flow into exercise 6.

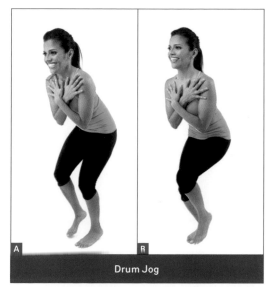

Drum Jog

6. Knee Raise Jog

FOCUS: Total body cardio

INTENTION: "I'm drumming a little louder now!"

GET IN POSITION: Begin by standing with your feet hip-width apart. Keep your feet parallel, with your toes in front of your heels. Raise your right knee at a 90-degree angle in front of and in line with your right hip. Keep your right foot flexed. Point your tailbone down. Tighten your abs by pulling your belly button in toward your spine. Stand tall as you lengthen

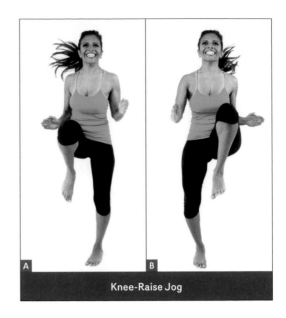

Knee-Raise Jog

your abs and chest up and away from your hips. Keep your chest open, with your shoulders back and down, away from your ears. Bend your arms at a 90-degree angle, palms facing in toward your body. Keep your head in line with your spine. Focus forward.

GET MOVING: Start jogging by dropping your right knee and right foot down to the floor as you lift your left knee up at a 90-degree angle in front of and in line with your left hip. Keep your body straight and steady as you hop back and forth, alternating your bent knees up and down. Keep your arms hugged into your body at 90-degree angles as you switch your knees fast. The goal is to get your knees up and across from your hip each time while keeping your arms and abs steady. Move with precision—act as if you have to stay in the same exact spot every time you move. Engage your core and increase your tempo.

SERIES: 30-second jog (Do as many knee raises in form as you can.)

LOOK OUT FOR: Moving too slowly. (The idea is to keep the heart rate up!) Not staying steady and maintaining tight rhythm.

NEED TO MODIFY? Tender knees or back: Do Standing March (p. 169) instead.

TRANSITION: Immediately round forward, place your hands on the floor, and step your legs back; flow into exercise 7. (Note: Let your breath come back to you while you set up your Plank.)

7. Plank Spidermans

FOCUS: Core and shoulders

INTENTION: "My core is steady as I climb to my limits."

GET IN POSITION: Begin in Plank position with your hands in line with your shoulders, palms flat and fingertips spread. Keep your feet hip-width apart. Straighten your legs. Tip your heels forward, as if you are stretching your feet and your body is about to take off. Level your hips and keep your back flat. Tighten your abs by pulling your belly button in toward your spine. Tuck your hips slightly so your back feels protected. Keep your chest open, with your shoulders back and down, away from your ears. Your head should be in line with your spine. Focus on the floor. Your entire body should feel solid, as if you're stuck in a tube.

GET MOVING: Continue to monitor the flatness of your body. Push away from the floor while maintaining good posture. Maintain straight legs. Keeping your left leg straight, bring your right knee out and up toward your right shoulder and then lower it back to center. (You will look like Spiderman going up a building!) Repeat the movement on your left side. Make sure to keep the leg that is not moving straight. Keep your chest open and your head in line with your spine. Keep shifting your weight forward slightly.

SERIES: 5-second hold 10 single count knee raises *right/center/left/center* (Tempo is key!) 10-second hold

LOOK OUT FOR: Keeping your hips too low or too high and arching or rounding your back as a result. Dropping your head. Rounding your shoulders. Placing your hands too close together or too far apart. Placing your hands too far forward and not in line with your shoulders. Not really bringing your knee forward to the fullest range possible. Arching your back instead of engaging your abs and tucking your hips slightly. Forgetting to tip your heels forward.

NEED TO MODIFY? Tender wrists or tight shoulders: Do Forearm Plank (p. 66) instead *or* skip bringing your knees up. Tender back: Give yourself mini-breaks and be patient.

TRANSITION: Come to your hands and knees and take a quick breath; flow into exercise 8.

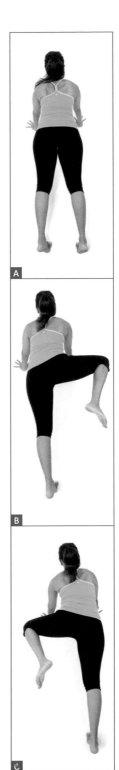

Plank Spidermans

8. Push-Up Spidermans

FOCUS: Chest, arms, and core

INTENTION: "Even if it is tiny, it counts—and I'm getting stronger."

GET IN POSITION: Begin in Plank position with your hands wider than your shoulders, palms flat and fingertips spread. Keep your feet hip-width apart. Straighten your legs. Tip your heels forward, as if you are stretching your feet and your body is about to take off. Level your hips and keep your back flat. Tighten your abs by pulling your belly button in toward your spine. Tuck your hips slightly so your back feels protected. Keep your chest open, with your shoulders back and down, away from your ears. Your head should be in line with your spine. Focus on the floor. Your entire body should feel solid, as if you're stuck in a tube.

GET MOVING: Keeping your left leg straight, bring your right knee out and up toward your right shoulder and then lower it back to center. Repeat the movement on your left side. After the right and left knee raises, do a push-up by bending your elbows, lowering your entire body to the floor, and then straightening your arms to lift your entire body back up. Leading with your chest, lower as far as you can without sacrificing your form— even a mini push-up counts! Make sure you keep tipping your heels forward with every push-up. Maintain good posture and tap into your core strength for this workout.

SERIES: 10 single count Spiderman push-ups (right and left knee raises followed by a push-up) 10 single count push-ups, *down/up*

LOOK OUT FOR: Keeping your hips too low or too high and arching or rounding your back as a result. Dropping your head. Rounding your shoulders. Placing your hands

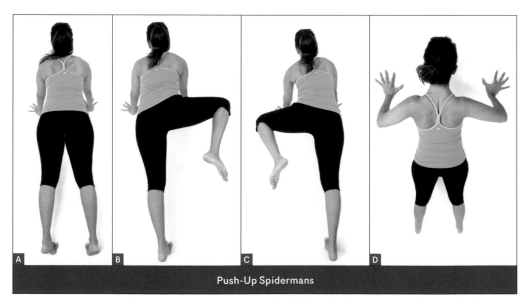

Push-Up Spidermans

too close together or too far apart. Placing your hands too far forward and not in line with your shoulders. Not bringing your knees close enough to your shoulders. Moving too fast. Arching your back instead of engaging your abs and tucking your hips slightly. Forgetting to tip your heels forward

NEED TO MODIFY? Tender wrists or tight shoulders: Make fists and substitute them for your flat palms. Tender back: Give yourself mini-breaks and be patient *or* do Push-Up Bent Knees (p. 88) instead.

TRANSITION: Come to your knees, shift your weight and rest back; flow into exercise 9.

9. Child's Pose with Arm Extension

FOCUS: Shoulders and chest

BREATHING TECHNIQUE: Inhale your arms up and forward toward head/Exhale your lower back and hips down.

GET IN POSITION: Begin by kneeling on the floor and sitting on your heels. Your feet should be comfortably together, with your knees apart and wider than your hips. Fold your upper body forward between your thighs and bring your forehead to the floor.

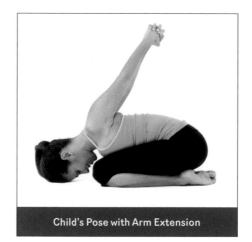

Child's Pose with Arm Extension

Clasp your hands together behind your back and reach your arms straight up toward the ceiling and forward toward your head. Rock your arms from side to side.

SERIES: 10-second hold

NEED TO MODIFY? Tender knees: Place a pillow under your hamstrings for elevation *or* play around with the placement of your knees until you feel comfortable.

TRANSITION: Roll your body up and bring your legs out in front of you; flow into exercise 10.

10. Tricep Dips

FOCUS: Triceps

INTENTION: "Let me train myself to feel the targeted triceps and not give up."

GET IN POSITION: Begin by sitting on the floor with your hands placed comfortably behind your back. Bend your knees at a 90-degree angle, keeping your feet flat on the floor. Your hands should be placed on the floor right under your shoulders, hugging your hips. Turn your palms out at a 90-degree angle. Keep your palms flat and spread

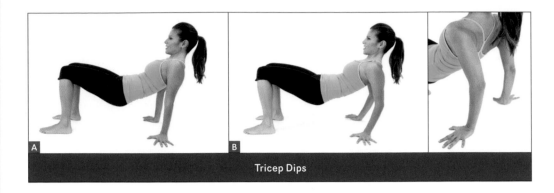

Tricep Dips

your fingertips. Lean back and press into your feet and hands to lift your hips up from the floor. Balance on your hands and feet, as you straighten your arms and press your hips up to be level with your knees and shoulders. Shift your body back into your hands again, aligning your shoulders slightly behind your wrists.

GET MOVING: Bend your elbows down to the floor and toward one another and then straighten your arms to lift back up. Try to keep your hips up and the rest of your body steady as you bend and drop your elbows only. Zero in and isolate just your triceps to do the work.

SERIES: 10 single count, *down/up* 10 pulses, *down/down* 10 single count, *down/up*

LOOK OUT FOR: Dropping your hips instead of just your elbows. Not leaning back into your hands. Letting your elbows bend out to the sides instead of in toward one another. Misplacing your palms, either not turning them out enough or turning them in too much.

NEED TO MODIFY? Tender wrists: Stay seated and bend your elbows. (Skip lifting up your hips.) Tight shoulders: Place your hands wider apart.

TRANSITION: Lie back and bring your legs and arms up; flow into exercise 11.

11. Stationary Bicycle Ab Series

FOCUS: Core

INTENTION: "This is supposed to be tough; I want things challenging and effective. I'm going to let go of any ego; I will strive for proper form as opposed to feeling pressure to be too advanced."

GET IN POSITION: Begin by lying flat on your back with your legs straight and feet hip-width apart. Lift your right leg and bend your right knee at a 90-degree angle. Get your right knee in line with your right hip and your right foot across from your knee; point your toes. Point your left toes and keep your left leg straight as you lift it up across from your left hip. Curl and round your upper body off the floor to clasp your hands and interlace your fingers behind your right knee. Keep your elbows wide and your shoulders down as you hollow out your upper body. Engage your abs by pulling them in tightly and scooping your hips up. (Create the letter "C" with your body.) Try to draw your chest up toward your knee. (Note: Your knee doesn't come to you; you curl up to your knee!) Press your lower back into the floor. Keep your head in line with your spine. Focus forward.

GET MOVING: Curl your upper body up toward your bent right knee. Use your arm strength to help you curl, keeping your elbows wide. Maintain a focused eye level and keep your legs stationary. (Don't let your feet/legs drop!) Create a deeper C with your back by pulling your belly in, grounding your lower back, and pulling your shoulders down. Keep all movements small. (Don't read into a small range of motion.) When curling, you should feel that you hit a wall with each curl. That "wall" is you pulling your abs tight. Let go with your hands only if you're ready! When letting go, straighten your arms with your palms facing down and try to maintain the same eye focus. If your upper body and eye level drop too much when you let go, it's not worth letting go!

SERIES: 5-second hold 10 single count, *up/down* 10 single count *up/down* release curls (Release arms to sides and curl.)* 10 single count *out/in* release taps behind knee (Release arms, make fists and tap in and out behind your bent knee.)* Quickly switch legs and repeat the series with your left leg bent and your right leg straight.

*Don't feel pressure to let go. Master holding on because that builds your strength most effectively. If letting go makes you feel unstable and/or lose form, it's not worth it. Do the same series holding on and try to keep your legs and upper body stable.

LOOK OUT FOR: Rounding your shoulders too much. Bringing your knee into your chest instead of your chest up toward your knee. Staying too low and using your neck to pull forward. Using your shoulders instead of your abs to lift your upper body. Not keeping your bottom straight leg engaged and off the floor. Being too ambitious with releasing your arms. Forgetting to breathe!

NEED TO MODIFY? Weak abs: Keep holding on with both hands. Back or hip issues: Keep your feet on the floor and continue. Tightness in neck or shoulders: Put a towel under your leg and hold onto the towel instead of your thigh.

TRANSITION: Sit up and place your hands flat on the floor; flow into exercise 12.

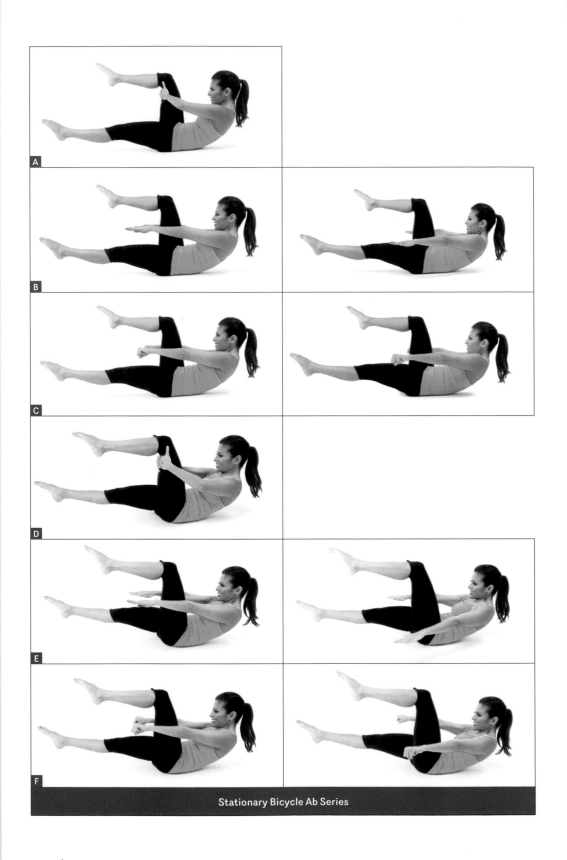

Stationary Bicycle Ab Series

12. Tricep Dip with Twisting Claps

FOCUS: Triceps

INTENTION: "Let me have fun the way a kid would, isolating my triceps and not giving up."

GET IN POSITION: Begin by sitting on the floor with your hands placed comfortably behind your back. Bend your knees at a 90-degree angle, keeping your feet flat on the floor. Your hands should be placed under your shoulders, hugging your hips. Turn your palms out at a 90-degree angle. Keep your palms flat and spread your fingertips. Lean back and press into your feet and hands to lift your hips up from the floor. Balance on your hands and feet, as you straighten your arms and press your hips up to be level with your knees and shoulders. Shift your weight back into your hands again, aligning your shoulders slightly behind your wrists.

GET MOVING: Bend your elbows down to the floor and toward one another and then straighten your arms to lift back up. After a down/up, balance on your right hand (right arm straight) and twist your left hand up to an extended right leg. After the twist, place your hand and foot back down into their original positions. Repeat the movement on the other side: lower *down/up* and then balance on your left hand with your (left arm straight) and twist your right hand up to an extended left leg. Try to keep your hips up and the rest of your body steady as you only bend and drop your elbows during the down/up. Zero in on and isolate just your triceps to do the work. Trust your body during the balance and really twist and try to reach and tap your hand as high as possible on the opposing leg (All the way up to the pointed toes if you can!)

SERIES: 20 Sets **Set:** 1 single count *down/up/twist left hand to tap straight right leg/drop left hand and right leg down* and then 1 single count *down/up/twist right hand to tap straight left leg/drop right hand and left leg down*

LOOK OUT FOR: Dropping your hips instead of just your elbows. Not leaning back into your hands. Letting your elbows bend out to the sides instead of in toward one another. Misplacing your palms, either not turning them out enough or turning them in too much. Bending your elbows on the twist.

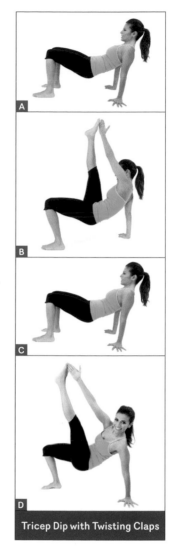

Tricep Dip with Twisting Claps

HAPPINESS

NEED TO MODIFY? Tender wrists: Stay seated and bend your elbows without lifting your hips *or* skip the twists. Tight shoulders: Place your hands wider apart.

TRANSITION: Lie back and bring your legs and arms up; flow into exercise 13.

13. Twisting Bicycle Ab Series

FOCUS: Core

INTENTION: "This is supposed to be tough; I want things challenging and effective. I'm going to let go of any ego; I will strive for proper form as opposed to feeling pressure to be too advanced."

GET IN POSITION: Begin by lying flat on your back with your legs straight and feet hip-width apart. Lift your right leg and bend your right knee at a 90-degree angle. Get your right knee in line with your right hip and your right foot across from your knee; point your toes. Point your left toes and keep your left leg straight as you lift it up in line with your left hip. Engage your abs by pulling them in tightly and press your lower back into the floor. Clasp your hands and interlace your fingers behind your head. It should feel as if your head is resting in a "pillow" of your hands. Keep your elbows wide. (Note: Move through the series swiftly; don't take too long of a break between sets!)

GET MOVING: Twist and curl your left elbow and shoulder toward your bent right knee and then alternate legs and twist the other way. Twist side to side with your upper body while switching bent legs. Use your core strength to help you curl. Keep your legs in precise form, don't let your knees fall in toward your chest.

SERIES: 20 sets **Set:** 1 single count twist (left elbow/shoulder to right knee) and then 1 single count twist (right elbow/shoulder to left knee)

LOOK OUT FOR: Moving with momentum instead of strength. Using your hip flexors instead of your core strength. Twisting with your elbow instead of your obliques. Overextending and stressing your neck to reach your shoulder toward the opposing knee. Bringing your knee into your chest instead of your chest up toward your knee. Not keeping your bottom straight leg engaged and off the floor. Forgetting to breathe!

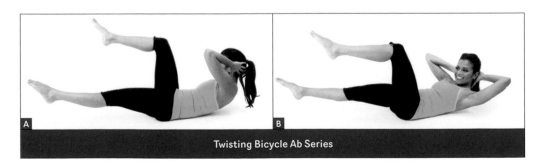

Twisting Bicycle Ab Series

NEED TO MODIFY? Weak abs: Do Stationary Bicycle Ab Series (p. 178) instead. Back or hip issues: Keep your feet on the floor and continue. Tightness in neck or shoulders: Do Crunch Series (p. 96) instead.

TRANSITION: Lie back and flip over onto your stomach; flow into exercise 14.

14. Cobra

FOCUS: Core and back

BREATHING TECHNIQUE: Inhale your chest up/Exhale your hips forward and shoulders back.

GET IN POSITION: Begin by lying on your stomach, propped on your forearms. Slide your hands back under your shoulders, keeping your palms flat and fingertips spread. Keep your elbows bent, hugging them tightly into your body. Keep your feet and knees hip-width apart. Press the tops

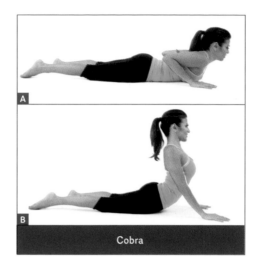

Cobra

of your feet, thighs, and hips firmly into the floor. Start to lengthen and straighten your arms while lifting your chest off the floor. Keep your shoulder blades back, puffing your ribs forward. Keep your hips connected to the floor and lift your upper body. (You might not be able to straighten your arms entirely, so feel free to keep your elbows slightly bent for comfort.) Firm up your butt and drive your hips forward while lifting your chest and stretching your abs. Twist your upper body to the right and to the left, lengthening your sides, and then return to center. (Repeat the movement twice.)

SERIES: 10-second hold

NEED TO MODIFY? Tender back: Do Cat/Cow (p. 99) instead.

TRANSITION: Stay lying down; flow into exercise 15.

15. Beach Bum Leg Lifts

FOCUS: Glutes, hamstrings, and inner thighs

INTENTION: "It's as if I'm at the beach and the sun is shining on my back as I enjoy getting a great workout for my butt just lying here!"

GET IN POSITION: Begin by lying on your stomach, resting your forehead on your hands. Keep your feet and knees hip-width apart. Lift and flex your right foot as you draw it toward your butt, creating a 90-degree angle with your leg and engaging your hamstring.

Engage and straighten your left leg as you point your left toes. Tuck your hips slightly. Tighten your abs by pulling your belly button in toward your spine.

GET MOVING: Maintain a flat back while you lift your right knee and leg up and down. Except for your right thigh, keep your entire body grounded (especially your hips). Try to keep your knee slightly above hip level. (Not too high or too low—slightly off the floor.) Engage your hamstring by pulling your right heel toward your butt. Constantly monitor your hips, tucking them forward slightly and protecting your back against the working leg trying to lift. Repeat the movement on your left side.

SERIES: 20 single count, *up/down* 20 pulses, *up/up* 20 multi-count, *up/up/up/down* 10 single count, *up/down* 10 pulses, *up/up* 5-second hold Rest (a couple of seconds; not too long!) and switch legs, repeating the same series on your left side.

LOOK OUT FOR: Arching your back. Forgetting to square off and ground your hips. Swinging your leg, as opposed to making a controlled movement. Keeping your leg too low, or not bringing your leg high enough.

NEED TO MODIFY? Tender back: Make very small movements and take breaks.

TRANSITION: Flip over; flow into exercise 16.

16. Heels Up Tucks

FOCUS: Glutes, hips, and inner thighs

INTENTION: "I can have fun right now."

GET IN POSITION: Begin by lying flat on your back. Bend your knees and draw your feet toward your butt, keeping your feet flat on the floor. Keep your feet wider than your hips. Walk your toes back an inch to raise your heels all the way up (as if you are wearing a pair of high heels). (Feel free to play around with your foot placement, closer together or farther apart, to get comfortable.) Turn your knees in slightly.

Beach Bum Leg Lifts

GET MOVING: Engage your abs by pulling them in tightly and grounding your back down into the floor. Tucking your pelvis under, press just your butt up and down off the floor. (Try to find a good beat with your butt lifts, like you're bouncing a basketball.) Maintain a small range of motion. (Less is more!) Make sure to keep your abs engaged and your back flat as you isolate just your butt to lift your hips. You're flipping your hips up toward your chest, doing a mini-lift with your butt. Keep your heels up high.

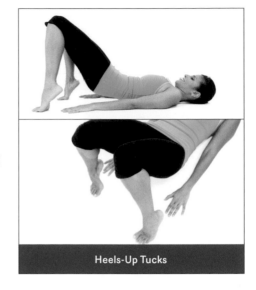

Heels-Up Tucks

SERIES: 20 single count, *up/down* 20 multi-count, *up/up/up/down* 20 single count, *up/down* 20 multi-count, *up/up/up/down* 10 single count, *up/down* 5-second hold

LOOK OUT FOR: Using your whole back to lift just your butt up. (Your back should not be off the floor.) Swinging your hips too high off the floor. Placing your feet too close to your butt. (Be nice to your knees!)

NEED TO MODIFY? Tender knees: Flex your feet instead of keeping your heels up.

TRANSITION: Stay on the floor; flow into exercise 17.

17. Lying 4 Stretch (Right/Left)

FOCUS: Glutes

BREATHING TECHNIQUE: Inhale your left knee into your chest/Exhale your right knee away from your chest as you lower your back to the floor. Inhale your right knee into your chest/Exhale your left knee away from your chest as you lower your back to the floor.

GET IN POSITION: Begin by lying flat on your back with your legs bent at a 90-degree angle and your feet flat on the floor. Lift your right leg up and gently place your right ankle on top of your left thigh, close to your left knee. Flex your foot. Lift your left foot off the floor as you draw your knees and legs in toward your chest. Flex your foot. Thread your arms through your legs, interlacing your fingers behind your left leg. Use your right elbow (or hand) to help you press and turn your right knee and thigh away from your body as you draw your left knee and thigh in toward your body. Press your butt down toward the floor while continuing to draw your left knee in. Repeat the movement on your left side.

SERIES: 10-second hold, right side (right ankle to left thigh) 10-second hold, left side (left ankle to right thigh)

NEED TO MODIFY? Tight hips or back: Keep the foot of your bottom leg on the floor instead of lifting it toward your chest.

TRANSITION: Hug your knees into your chest; flow into exercise 18.

18. Back Rolls/Circle

FOCUS: Back and core

BREATHING TECHNIQUE: Inhale to hug your knees and roll your back down/Exhale to hug knees and roll your back up. Play around: Maybe try 10 full circles, as if you are mimicking the hands on a clock. The point is having fun and rolling!

GET IN POSITION: Begin by lying flat on your back, hugging your knees into your chest comfortably. (How much space is between your knees depends on your flexibility and comfort.) Wrap your arms around your legs. Option: Hold your shins or arms or even your wrists. (Your hand placement depends on flexibility and comfort.) Keep your toes pointed. Engage your abs and swing your feet a little as you roll your body all the way up to balance and sit on your butt and roll back down to your original position.

SERIES: 10 breaths, *inhale/exhale* (10 roll-ups/10 roll-downs) Make sure to take long, full breaths.

NEED TO MODIFY? Tender back: Skip rolling and lift and lower your knees into and away from your chest.

TRANSITION: Bring your body up to a seated position on the last roll and sit on your feet; flow into exercise 19.

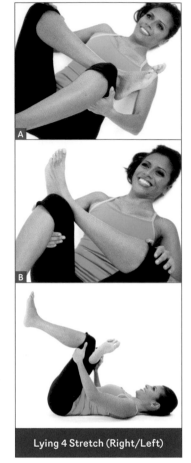

Lying 4 Stretch (Right/Left)

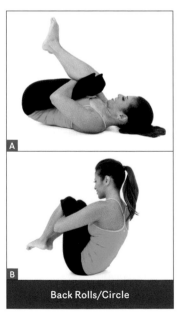

Back Rolls/Circle

19. Knee Dancing

FOCUS: Thighs

INTENTION: "Wow! This burns and is hard. Thank goodness I'm happy, and I can handle it!"

GET IN POSITION: Begin by kneeling on the floor and sitting on your heels. Your feet should be comfortably together, with your knees apart and wider than your hips. Toes should be behind your heels. Lean back as you line your shoulders up with your hips. Tighten your abs by pulling your belly button in toward your spine. Tuck your hips slightly, scooping your butt forward. Extend and straighten your arms above your head, toward the ceiling. Interlock your thumbs and face your palms forward. Lengthen your abs and chest up and away from your hips. Continue to reach your arms up as you push your shoulders down. Maintain good posture and keep leaning back. (Avoid the temptation to lean forward.) Your head should be in line with your spine. Focus forward.

GET MOVING: Using the strength of your thighs, lift your butt about 1 inch above your feet. (Only an inch; it is tempting to go too high!) Lean back and keep aligning your shoulders with your heels and your hands with your head. Make this your "sweet spot" and move into the series from there. (Try to hover above your feet the entire time.) You have

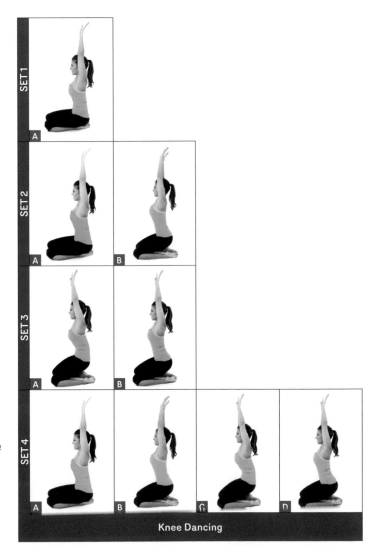

Knee Dancing

to remind yourself to keep these movements small and lean back constantly. (This can be really hard to do!)

SERIES: Set 1: *Hold* Lift your butt 1 inch above your heels and hold. 10-second hold Rest (a couple of seconds; not too long!) Set 2: *Lifts* Lift your butt 1 inch above your heels and move up an inch and down an inch from there. 10 single count, *up/down* 5-second hold Rest (a couple of seconds; not too long!) Set 3: *Tucks* Lift your butt 1 inch above your heels and tuck your hips forward and back from there. 10 single count tucks *up/back* 5-second hold Rest (a couple of seconds; not too long!) Set 4: *Lift/Tuck Combo* Lift your butt 1 inch above your heels and combine the sets from before. 10 single count lifts *up/down* 10 single count tucks *up/back* 5-second hold

LOOK OUT FOR: Leaning your upper body too far forward. Lifting your butt too high off your feet. (It's easier that way, but we don't want that!)

NEED TO MODIFY? Knee issues: Do Seated Leg lifts (p. 91) instead. Foot cramps: Curl your toes under instead of keeping your feet flat and toes pointed.

TRANSITION: Place your hands down and lean back; flow into exercise 20.

20. Double Thigh Stretch

FOCUS: Thighs

BREATHING TECHNIQUE: Inhale your hips up and butt forward/Exhale, bend your elbows, and lean back.

GET IN POSITION: Begin by kneeling on the floor and sitting on your heels. Your feet should be comfortably together, with your knees apart and wider than your hips. Place your palms on the floor behind your feet. (Choose a range that is comfortable and turn your hands out for wrist comfort.) Lean back into your hands while lifting your hips and squeezing your butt up. Bend your elbows back as you try to maintain the space between your butt and feet.

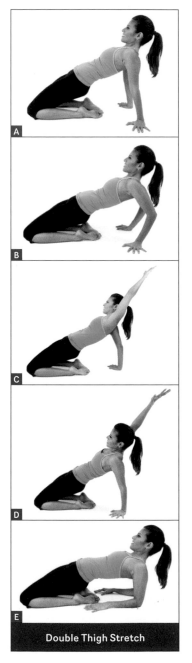

Double Thigh Stretch

SERIES: 5-second hold (Bend your elbows straight back.) 5-second hold, right side (Left arm reaches toward right side.) 5-second hold, left side (Right arm reaches toward left side.) 5-second hold, center (Bend your elbows as low as you can.)

NEED TO MODIFY? Tender knees: Lie on your right side and bend your left knee. Reach your left arm behind you to grab your left foot with your left hand. Bend your left elbow as you squeeze your hips and butt forward. Repeat on the other side.

TRANSITION: Step your right leg forward; flow into exercise 21.

21. Hip Flexor Stretch (Left)

FOCUS: Hip flexor

BREATHING TECHNIQUE: Inhale your left hip forward/Exhale your right hip back. Inhale your abs in and up/Exhale your upper body back.

GET IN POSITION: Begin with your right leg in front in lunge position, with your right knee over your right heel. Keep your left leg parallel and on the ground, with your left foot in line with your left hip. Turn your left hip forward and make sure your hips are squared. Tuck your hips forward as you lift your abs and chest up and away from your hips. Reach your arms up straight up toward the ceiling. Keep your palms facing in. Tighten your abs by pulling your belly button in toward your spine. Lean your upper body back. Keep your chest open, with your shoulders back and down, away from your ears. Your head should be in line with your spine. Focus forward.

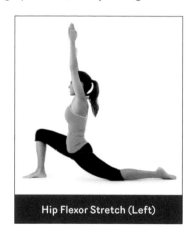

Hip Flexor Stretch (Left)

SERIES: 10-second hold

NEED TO MODIFY? Tight hips: Keep your hands on the floor on either side of your front foot.

TRANSITION: Stay in position and swiftly take your right hand back; flow into exercise 22.

22. Single Thigh Stretch (Left)

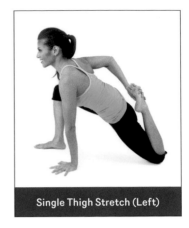

Single Thigh Stretch (Left)

FOCUS: Thighs

BREATHING TECHNIQUE: Inhale and lift your abs and chest up/Exhale and squeeze your hips forward and pull your foot toward your butt.

GET IN POSITION: Begin with your right leg in front in lunge position, with your right knee over your right heel. Keep your left leg parallel and on the ground, with your left foot in line with your left hip. Turn your left hip forward and make sure your hips are squared. Reach your left arm straight down to the floor and try to flatten your palm. Bend your left knee, drawing your back foot off the floor. Take your right hand back, and grab your left foot; point your toes. Bend your right elbow more, pulling your left foot closer to your hips. Lean your upper body back as your butt and hips squeeze forward. Tighten your abs by pulling your belly button in toward your spine. Lengthen your abs and chest up and away from your hips as you pull your foot up. Keep your chest open, with your shoulders back and down, away from your ears. Your head should be in line with your spine. Focus forward.

SERIES: 10-second hold

NEED TO MODIFY? Unable to grab foot: Use a towel and wrap it around your ankle to help.

TRANSITION: Lower your leg and step back; flow into exercise 23.

23. Down Dog

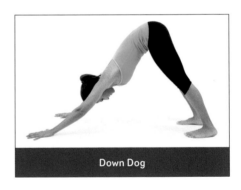

Down Dog

FOCUS: Hamstrings and back

BREATHING TECHNIQUE: Inhale your arms long and hips up/Exhale your shoulders down and heels toward the floor.

GET IN POSITION: Begin in Plank position with your hands in line with your shoulders, palms flat and fingertips spread. Your palms (parallel or slightly turned out) should be flat and your fingers spread. Keep your toes curled as you shift your weight back and lift your hips up toward the ceiling. As you start to lengthen your arms and legs, continue to press your palms and heels down. As your hips rise toward the ceiling, push the tops of your thighs back and stretch your heels down to the floor, lengthening your hamstrings. Straighten your knees but do not lock them. Maintain straight legs. (Soften your knees if your lower back or hamstrings are tight.) Rotate your elbows in to firm up the arms and shoulders. Maintain a long back. Keep your head in line with your arms; do not hang your head down. (Note: Imagine you're creating a teepee with your body!)

SERIES: 10-second hold

NEED TO MODIFY? Tender knees or tight back and hamstrings: Keep your legs bent and heels raised.

TRANSITION: Step your left leg forward; flow into exercise 24.

24. Hip Flexor Stretch (Right)

Repeat exercise 21 with your left leg forward.

TRANSITION: Stay in position and swiftly take your left hand back; flow into exercise 25.

25. Single Thigh Stretch (Right)

Repeat exercise 22 with your left leg forward.

TRANSITION: Lower your leg and step back; flow into exercise 26.

26. Down Dog

Repeat exercise 23.

TRANSITION: Rest your knees down and lean your upper body back; flow into exercise 27.

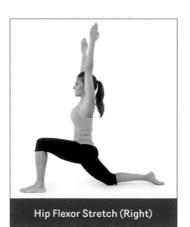

Hip Flexor Stretch (Right)

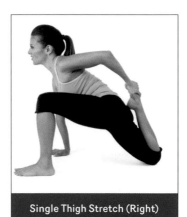

Single Thigh Stretch (Right)

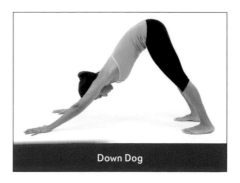

Down Dog

27. Kneeling Meditation

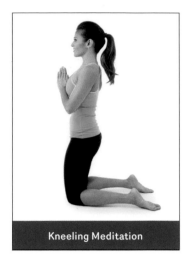

Kneeling Meditation

FOCUS: Total body awareness

MANTRA: Thank you.

BREATHING TECHNIQUE: Inhale your chest up/Exhale your shoulders back. Embrace your gratitude.

GET IN POSITION: Kneel on the floor with your knees hip-width apart. Keep your legs parallel behind you with your toes pointed. Point your tailbone down. Tighten your abs by pulling your belly button in toward your spine. Lift your upper body toward the ceiling, as you lengthen your abs and chest up and away from your hips. Keep your chest open, with your shoulders back and down, away from your ears. Your head should be in line with your spine. Focus forward. Bring your palms together in front of your chest.

SERIES: 30-second hold or longer

NEED TO MODIFY? Close your eyes to help you focus better.

THE POST-WORKOUT

1 **Post-Workout Recap:**

You deserve an extra-high five, not only for the happy recognition that led you here, but also for the happy workout you can add to your roster of accomplishments. Sometimes it's hard to focus when all you want to do is sing out to the world and celebrate that you're in such a great mood. Instead, you took the time to truly reflect on the source of your happiness and channel that appreciation toward a joy-filled workout.

Did my emotional weight change?

☐ YES   ☐ NO

Did I accomplish my workout intention?

☐ YES   ☐ NO

Is there a change in my physical body?

☐ YES   ☐ NO

2 **My Post-Workout Mood Is:**

(Write down, think, or say out loud.)

_____

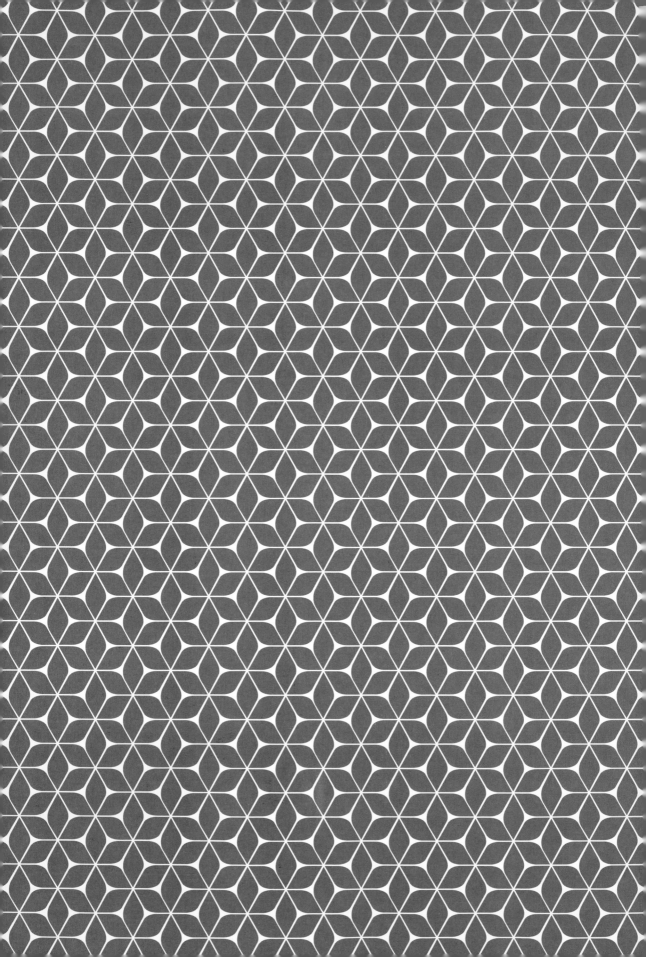

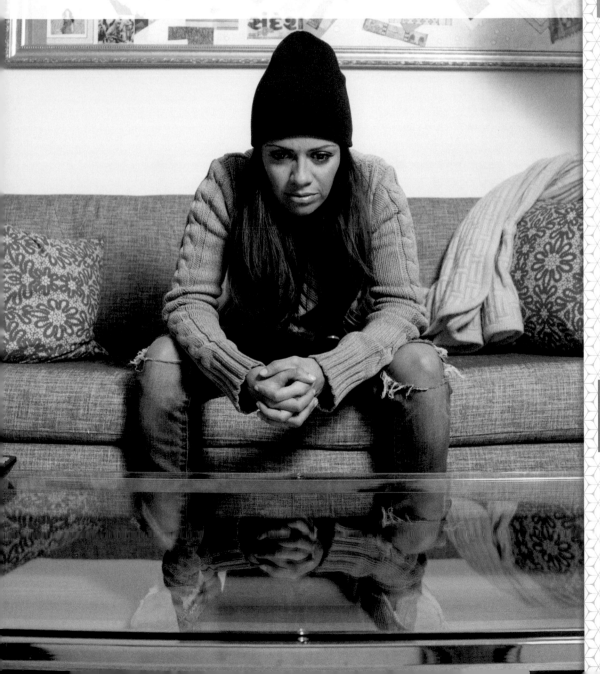

CHAPTER 8 —
THE DOUBT WORKOUT

THE DOUBT EXERCISES

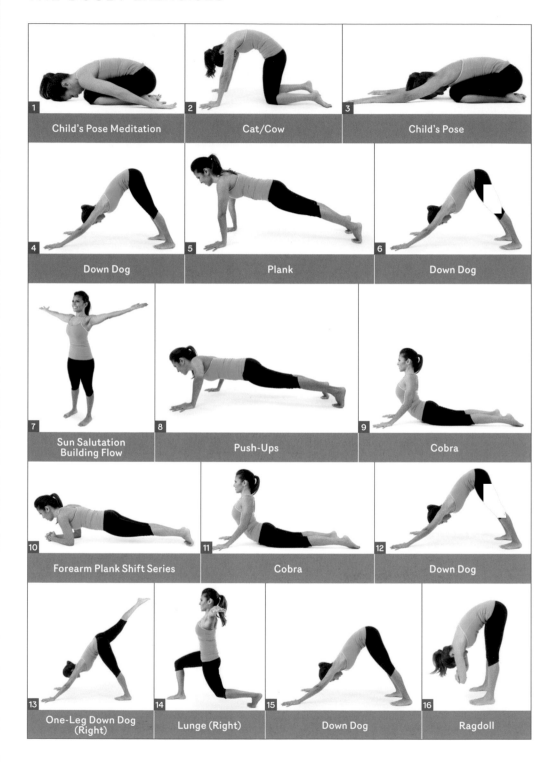

1. Child's Pose Meditation
2. Cat/Cow
3. Child's Pose
4. Down Dog
5. Plank
6. Down Dog
7. Sun Salutation Building Flow
8. Push-Ups
9. Cobra
10. Forearm Plank Shift Series
11. Cobra
12. Down Dog
13. One-Leg Down Dog (Right)
14. Lunge (Right)
15. Down Dog
16. Ragdoll

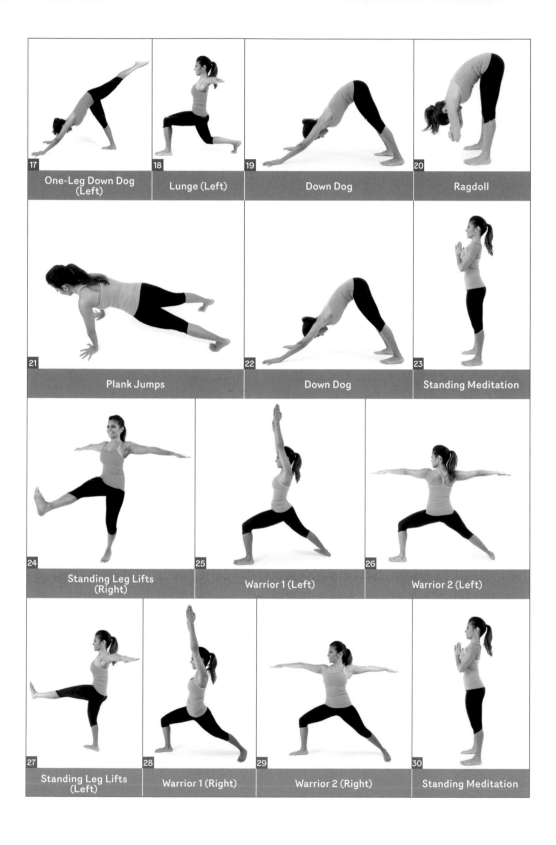

17 One-Leg Down Dog (Left)

18 Lunge (Left)

19 Down Dog

20 Ragdoll

21 Plank Jumps

22 Down Dog

23 Standing Meditation

24 Standing Leg Lifts (Right)

25 Warrior 1 (Left)

26 Warrior 2 (Left)

27 Standing Leg Lifts (Left)

28 Warrior 1 (Right)

29 Warrior 2 (Right)

30 Standing Meditation

Self-doubt is an emotion that can push you down with the weight of the universe, just like anger and anxiety. You'll see many of the descriptive words and physical symptoms overlap. What might help you pinpoint your mood/workout more precisely is to think of anger and anxiety as moods that are often triggered by external circumstances: Your boss yelled at you for something you didn't do; your taxi got a flat tire on the way to the airport and you're frantic you'll miss your plane. Doubt, however, tends to be more about self-criticism. Anger and anxiety are moods that are clear-cut and may end as soon as the situation is resolved: Your boss apologizes and gives you a raise; you are early for your plane and get upgraded. While doubt tends to linger . . . and linger . . . and just when you think it's gone, it can come back to taunt you, even in times of happiness or when you're feeling particularly grounded or accomplished. Doubt is the little voice we all have that says, "You'll never . . ." or, "You can't . . ."

And boy, those dot, dot, dots can get filled in awfully fast, can't they?

Is there one doubtful thought in particular that keeps you up at night? The special one that makes you feel self-critical and hopeless? The thought that is making you want to wring your hands, eat a pint of ice cream, or crawl into bed and put the covers over your head and never crawl back out again? What thought is stuck on replay? That is the thought I want you to own.

What is the emotional weight of that thought and its resulting mood, and how is it manifesting in your physical body?

THE PRE-WORKOUT

1 I Am Feeling:

☐ Angry	☐ Envious	☐ Indignant
☐ Annoyed	☐ Exasperated	☐ Intimidated
☐ Apathetic	☐ Fearful	☐ Irritated
☐ Confused	☐ Frustrated	☐ Jealous
☐ Crabby	☐ Grouchy	☐ Lonely
☐ Cranky	☐ Gullible	☐ Mean
☐ Dejected	☐ Hesitant	☐ Misgivings
☐ Demoralized	☐ Inadequate	☐ Mistrustful
☐ Disbelieving	☐ Incensed	☐ Mopey
☐ Discomfited	☐ Indecisive	☐ Morose
☐ Disgruntled	☐ Indifferent	☐ Petulant

☐ Provoking	☐ Sad	☐ Trepidation
☐ Qualms	☐ Skeptical	☐ Uncertain
☐ Quarrelsome	☐ Sulky	☐ Unclear
☐ Questioning	☐ Suppressed	☐ Uneasy
☐ Reservations	☐ Suspicious	☐ Worried
☐ Riled-Up	☐ Touchy	

Choose from the list above, or add your own words. Then write down *or* say your mood out loud, and embrace it.

2 **My Current Mood Is:**

_____

3 **My Emotional Weight Is:**

1	5	10
Light	Neutral	Heavy

4 **My Physical Symptoms Are:**

☐ Adrenaline Rush	☐ Head Rubbing	☐ Rapid Heartbeat
☐ Aggression	☐ Hot Flashes	☐ Shaking
☐ Clenching	☐ Heavy Breathing	☐ Stomachache
☐ Cramps	☐ Heavy Chest	☐ Sweating
☐ Crying	☐ Hunching	☐ Teeth Grinding
☐ Drooping	☐ Jaw Clenching	☐ Tightness
☐ Feeling Flushed	☐ Pacing	
☐ Fist Pounding	☐ Prickly Sensations	
☐ Goosebumps	☐ Raised Voice	

DOUBT

TEN COMMON **DOUBT** THOUGHTS

- I'll never be good enough.
- Why can't I lose weight? I feel fat and I'll always be fat.
- Why doesn't he love me?
- I'll never have the courage to ask for what I want.
- Why is it so easy for them when I just can't even come close to what they can do?
- Why do these things always happen to me? I'm like a magnet for distress.
- It's not gonna happen so why should I even try?
- Even if you said I was the best, I still wouldn't believe you.
- I just can't do it. I was born this way, I guess.
- Life is just so hard.

THE WORKOUT

1 Mantra for Doubt:

No one can take away your happiness.

Doubt sits heavily in a grey place for me. The uncertain nature of it gets me stuck in a circle, having the same thoughts over and over again, without an escape route.

I know logically that everyone has doubts, of course. Everyone wonders about their place in the world and if their life will play out according to their dreams. And everyone, even those who are seemingly the most successful, can be tortured by doubts in the still of the night. But when I'm in doubt, I feel so alone. As if I'm the only one who has or will ever experience my mood. But one day I truly realized that you're never alone in doubt. You've got your own worst enemy keeping you company and weighing you down . . . yourself!

I see this in my classes every day: women who are brimming with vitality; who are strong, flexible, and responsive to my workouts; who are slim and trim and look fantastic. They stare at themselves in the mirror with a despairing look (when they think I can't see them), and I know they're thinking, *I'm too fat. I'll never be skinny enough. I'll never do as many reps as so-and-so. I'll never have shiny hair like so-and-so. I'll never look as good in my workout gear as so-and-so. I'll never be in love. I'll never get married. I'll never be a mom. I'm just not good enough.*

It's at these times that their emotional weight is far heavier than their bodies will ever be. And it breaks my heart.

I wish I could bring my dad into class sometimes, so he could impart his wisdom to my clients as he does for me, in the hopes they will believe what he tells them too. Growing up, I saw disappointments in my father's life. Family took advantage of him, business partners stole from him, and he experienced death of loved ones, betrayal, and countless other challenging situations. And yet, without a hint of doubt in his delivery, he always proudly said, "I'm happy."

Hearing this, I felt the same disbelief as when I was told there were no problems in the world, only solutions. Was he lying? Was he in denial? Was he just trying to protect me? Was this his coping mechanism? *Where was his doubt?* I just didn't understand because it made me question my own feelings. I didn't always feel happy. Was there something wrong with me?

Given time and experience, I finally understood this lesson. I not only deeply believe my father when he says he is happy, but I also constantly and genuinely say it myself. I've learned how to push past my doubts and shut off that little nagging voice that wants so badly to tell me how much I messed up and will continue to mess up!

When I was nine years old, I was upset because I wasn't "cool" at school. I thought that if I only figured out how to achieve coolness, I would truly be happy.

"I'm not happy because those girls at school don't think I'm cool," I said to my dad.

"Honey, no one can take away your happiness," he quickly replied.

"What do you mean?" I retorted. "They already have. Maybe they don't want me to be happy. Maybe they really don't like me. I know I could be cool! I'm just *not*. I have to do something different."

"So you think if you change who you are you'll be happy?" he asked.

"Yes," I said defiantly. "I'll be more like them and we'll be friends. If I'm cool, I'll be happy and they'll be happy too!"

"Honey, you can't give away your happiness, either."

"But what if I want to?"

"You still can't."

"I do things that make you and Mommy happy, don't I?" I asked, frustrated.

"No. We make *ourselves* happy."

I went off to my room to cry, crushed by his harsh (yet truthful) words. How could my own father tell me that I didn't make him happy? I felt utterly powerless, insignificant, and confused about being happy ever again. (And I certainly would never be cool!) I knew my father truly loved me, but he was telling me that who I was and what I did didn't change him. I had always thought there was an easy solution for being happy and that I had a direct effect on others' happiness.

For my father, however, happiness and doubt were choices. A choice between embracing your ability to control the way you experience life, thereby allowing yourself to feel an entire range of emotions from the most ecstatically positive to the most painfully negative, and *not* embracing your ability to control the way you experience life, thereby *reacting* to both positive and negative emotions.

In other words, my father was telling me to take responsibility. He wanted me to own my moral compass and find the ability to point the magnetic needle due north, in the opposite direction of the doubts that were pulling me down.

Allowing myself to feel doubt or sadness versus *reacting* with doubt and sadness may seem like a subtle choice. But in my life, it's been the difference between happiness and unhappiness. Surrendering and accepting my emotions in order to more effectively express and release them is what helped me push past the doubts about being cool in school and move beyond the current doubts that creep up when I'm trying to complete a project or achieve a goal.

Let's couple the "No one can take away your happiness" mantra with the mantra from the Anger workout in Chapter 3, "The solution is born before the problem." Since a solution always exists and finding it is an ability we can choose to embrace, we can also say that no one can take away our ability to find solutions. So, if the ultimate solution is a life freed from chronic doubting, then no one can take away our ability to make the doubts less overwhelming. It's our decision and responsibility to chase away the doubts—and find that happiness.

My father knows that whatever happens, his *reaction* is up to him. He chooses to feel happy or unhappy. He was genuinely happy even after getting married without parental approval, coming to America with only $8, working three jobs, and losing all of his hard-earned money in a fire that burned down his first business. It's his resilience and unwillingness to surrender his own happiness to the outside world that have allowed him to create a life without doubt. Now I love it when he says, "Rupa, you are the captain of your soul and the driver of your own life. No one can take away your happiness." In my life, there will be obstacles, challenges, and doubts. With these consistent words and actions, I now feel a priceless sense of validation, freedom, and strength.

You can easily succumb to doubts or make the choice to flip them and be determined to point your mind and heart north. Since you can choose whether or not you ignore this power you have, try embracing it, so you can begin living the happiest, healthiest life possible.

2 **How to Use the Mantra**

When a toddler starts to walk, does he give up every time he falls? Of course not. Do we give up on him every time he falls? Of course not. He picks himself up and keeps trying and we stretch our hands out and encourage him. We pick him up and support him with the love, patience, and faith to try again and master walking across the living room. We act like his best friend, not his worst enemy. "No one can take away your happiness" is about becoming your own best friend. You were a toddler once and are fully capable of tapping into that loving perseverance again.

Repeat the "No one can take away your happiness" mantra and reclaim your power for a successful workout. If you believe you can do it, you can do it! Transforming your doubt into the ability to do a satisfying workout is incredibly empowering.

3 **Why the Doubt Workout**

By now you are very aware of what's triggering your doubts, and how they weigh you down emotionally and physically.

The flow of this exercise series is designed for you to slowly build your confidence back up and lift the weight of the world off your shoulders. As the workout develops, you will develop, as the physical challenges build your internal and external strength.

Embrace your mood, reflect on the mantra, and let it provide you with all the courage and stamina to make it through this mind and body-reassuring routine.

4 **My Doubt Workout Intention (Emotional or Physical) Is:**

(Write down, think, or say out loud.)

_____

MUSIC

Choose music that will empower you and make you feel more confident. Here are a few suggestions that will get the self-esteem flowing:

1960s: "Suspicious Minds" ▪ Elvis Presley

1970s: "I Will Survive" ▪ Gloria Gaynor

1980s: "I'm Coming Out" ▪ Diana Ross

1990s: "Vogue" ▪ Madonna

2000s: "Video" ▪ India Arie

2010s: "Roar" or "Firework" ▪ Katy Perry

THE DOUBT WORKOUT | 203

5 **The Doubt Exercises**

1. Child's Pose Meditation

FOCUS: Shoulders and back

MANTRA: No one can take away your happiness.

BREATHING TECHNIQUE: Inhale and exhale; observe your chest rising and falling. Embrace a sense of calm.

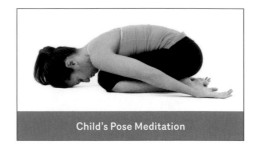

Child's Pose Meditation

GET IN POSITION: Begin by kneeling on the floor and sitting on your heels. Your feet should be comfortably together, with your knees apart and wider than your hips. Fold your upper body forward between your thighs and bring your forehead to the floor. Place your straight arms back alongside your torso with your palms up. Release your shoulders toward the floor.

SERIES: 10-second hold

NEED TO MODIFY? Tender knees: Place a pillow under your hamstrings for elevation *or* play around with the placement of your knees until you feel comfortable.

TRANSITION: Shift your weight forward onto your hands and knees; flow into exercise 2.

2. Cat/Cow

FOCUS: Core and back

BREATHING TECHNIQUE: Inhale fully into Cow/Exhale fully into Cat.

GET IN POSITION: Begin on all fours (on hands and knees) with your feet and knees hip-width apart. Your hands should be under your shoulders and your knees under your hips. Keep your hips squared. *Inhale into Cow:* Drop your belly and arch your back to bring your chest through your shoulders, moving your shoulders away from your ears. Your head and butt are reaching up toward the ceiling. *Exhale into*

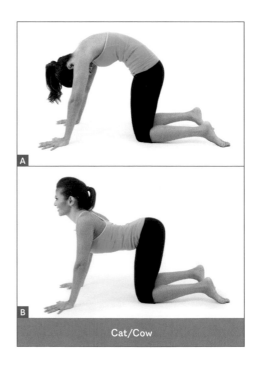

Cat/Cow

Cat: Round your back, drawing your belly up toward the ceiling. Drop your head toward the floor and tuck your hips.

SERIES: 3 breaths, *inhale/exhale* (3 Cows/3 Cats) Make sure to take long, full breaths.

NEED TO MODIFY? Tender knees: Fold your mat under your knees for extra cushioning. Tender neck: Avoid dropping your neck forward and pulling it back.

TRANSITION: Shift your weight and rest back; flow into exercise 3.

3. Child's Pose

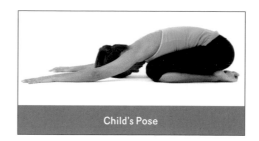

Child's Pose

FOCUS: Shoulders and back

MANTRA: No one can take away your happiness.

BREATHING TECHNIQUE: Inhale and exhale; observe your chest rising and falling. Embrace a sense of calm.

GET IN POSITION: Begin by kneeling on the floor and sitting on your heels. Your feet should be comfortably together, with your knees apart and wider than your hips. Fold your upper body forward between your thighs and bring your forehead to the floor. Reach your straight arms forward with your palms down. Release your shoulders toward the floor.

SERIES: 10-second hold

NEED TO MODIFY? Tender knees: Place a pillow under your hamstrings for elevation *or* play around with the placement of your knees until you feel comfortable.

TRANSITION: Shift your weight and hips back and up; flow into exercise 4.

4. Down Dog

FOCUS: Hamstrings and back

BREATHING TECHNIQUE: Inhale your arms long and hips up/Exhale your shoulders down and heels toward the floor.

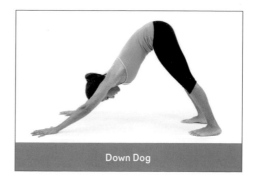

Down Dog

GET IN POSITION: Beginning in Cat/Cow position, make sure your hands are slightly in front of your shoulders. Your palms (parallel or slightly turned out) should be flat and your fingers spread. Curl your toes under and lift your knees and hips up. Start shifting your weight back and out of your shoulders. As you lengthen your arms and legs, continue to press your palms and heels down. As your hips rise toward the ceiling, push the tops of your thighs back and stretch your heels down to the floor, lengthening your hamstrings. Straighten your knees but do not lock them. Maintain straight legs. (Soften your knees if your lower back or hamstrings are tight.) Rotate your elbows in to firm up the arms and shoulders. Maintain a long back. Keep your head in line with your arms; do not hang your head down. (Note: Imagine you're creating a teepee with your body!)

SERIES: 10-second hold

NEED TO MODIFY? Tender knees or tight back and hamstrings: Keep your legs bent and heels raised.

TRANSITION: Shift your weight forward; flow into exercise 5.

5. Plank

FOCUS: Core and shoulders

INTENTION: "I can do this. Stay calm, and focus on the form."

GET IN POSITION: Begin on all fours (on hands and knees) with your feet and knees hip-width apart. Your hands should be in

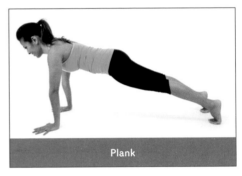
Plank

line with your shoulders, palms flat and fingertips spread. Curl your toes under to lift and straighten your legs. Tip your heels forward, as if you are stretching your feet and your body is about to take off. Level your hips and keep your back flat. Tighten your abs by pulling your belly button in toward your spine. Tuck your hips slightly so your back feels protected. Keep your chest open, with your shoulders back and down, away from your ears. Your head should be in line with your spine. Focus on the floor. Your entire body should feel solid, as if you're stuck in a tube.

GET MOVING: Continue to monitor the flatness of your body. Push away from the floor while maintaining good posture. Maintain straight legs. Keep your chest open and your head in line with your spine. Keep shifting your weight forward slightly.

SERIES: 1-minute hold

LOOK OUT FOR: Keeping your hips too low or too high and arching or rounding your back as a result. Dropping your head. Rounding your shoulders. Placing your hands too close together or too far apart. Placing your hands too far forward and not in line with your shoulders. Arching your back instead of engaging your abs and tucking your hips slightly. Forgetting to tip your heels forward.

NEED TO MODIFY? Tender wrists or tight shoulders: Do Forearm Plank (p. 66) instead. Tender back: Give yourself mini-breaks and be patient.

TRANSITION: Shift your weight and hips back and up; flow into exercise 6.

6. Down Dog

Repeat exercise 4.

TRANSITION: Walk your hands back and roll your body up; flow into exercise 7.

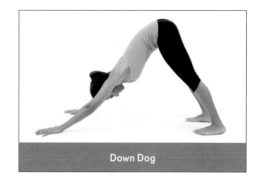
Down Dog

7. Sun Salutation Building Flow

FOCUS: Total body strength and flexibility

INTENTION: "I'm going to get more confident with each salutation."

GET IN POSITION: Be familiar with the Sun Salutation Basic Flow breakdown below. Breathing consciously is key to all Sun Salutations—make sure to take long, full breaths. Always link the motion of your breath to the movement of your body. The **boldface instructions (Step 6)** indicate where the degree of difficulty will increase each time in the series and what will make this Basic Flow "build." *Sun Salutation Basic Flow:* 1. Stand in Standing Meditation. 2. Sweep and raise your extended arms up toward the ceiling, palms facing and touching each other (inhale). 3. Turn your palms out, sweep your arms down, and bend at your waist into Standing Forward Bend (exhale). 4. Lift your upper body to a flat back (inhale). 5. Fold your body over again into Standing Forward Bend (exhale). 6. **Step back with your right leg and then your left leg, into Plank** (inhale). 7. Push into Down Dog; hold for 5 breaths (exhale). 8. Bend your right knee to step your right foot and then your left foot forward (inhale). 9. Adjust and try to flatten your palms against the floor in Standing Forward Bend (exhale). 10. Sweep and raise your extended arms up toward the ceiling, palms facing and touching each other (inhale). 11. Turn your palms out, sweep your arms down, and stand in Standing Meditation (exhale).

GET MOVING: Perform 3 Sun Salutations (from above) and increase the degree of difficulty each time by replacing **Step 6** with the direction from the series below.

SERIES: *Sun Salutation 1:* 10 single taps, *right/center/left/center* in Plank* *Sun Salutation 2:* 10 single taps, *right/center/left/center*, and 10 single count *bend/stretch* in Plank** *Sun Salutation 3:* 10 single combinations, *right/center/left/center/bend/stretch/down/up****

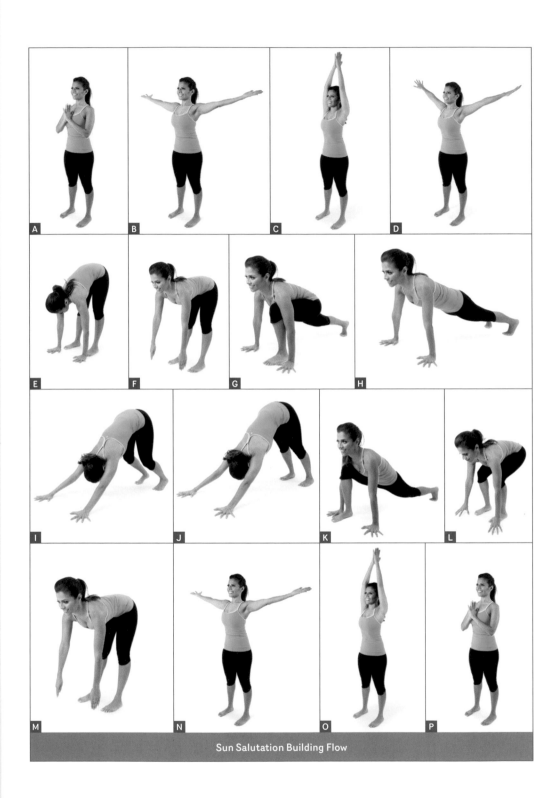

Sun Salutation Building Flow

Taps meaning: Maintaining a flat back and keeping your right leg straight, tap your right foot out to the right side and then bring it back to center. Repeat the movement on your left side. **Bend/stretch* meaning: Maintaining a flat back, bend and stretch just your knees and then straighten your legs. Make sure your bends are tiny as you keep the rest of your body solid. ***Think of it simply! You're combining the two different parts from Sun Salutation 2 with a push-up: tap your right and then left foot out once, bend and stretch your knees once, and then perform a push-up by lowering and raising your body once. Repeat 10 times. Cut your last salutation short by shifting into the Down Dog from your last Push-Up and staying there for 5 breaths, *inhale/exhale*.

LOOK OUT FOR: Rushing and forgetting to link your breath to your flow. Putting pressure on yourself to demonstrate more flexibility and strength. (This is really all about flow!) Keeping your hips too low or too high and arching or rounding your back as a result. Dropping your head. Rounding your shoulders. Placing your hands too close together or too far apart. Placing your hands too far forward and not in line with your shoulders. During taps: Bending your legs when tapping instead of keeping your legs straight. During bend/ stretch: Bending your knees too much and sacrificing the flatness of your back. Being bouncy in your movements instead of controlled. Arching your back instead of engaging your abs and tucking your hips slightly. Forgetting to tip your heels forward in Step 6.

NEED TO MODIFY? Tight hamstrings: Bend your knees in Standing Forward Bends. Too challenging: Slowly build as desired *or* stick with the Sun Salutation Basic Flow only.

TRANSITION: Shift your weight forward and place your hands wider, flow into exercise 8.

8. Push-Ups

FOCUS: Chest, arms, and core

INTENTION: "Even if it is tiny, it counts—and I'm getting stronger."

GET IN POSITION: Begin in Plank position with your hands wider than your shoulders, palms flat and fingertips spread. Keep your feet hip-width apart. Straighten your legs. Tip your heels forward, as if you are stretching your feet and your body is about to take off. Level your hips and keep your back flat. Tighten your abs by pulling your belly button in toward your spine. Tuck your hips slightly so your back feels protected.

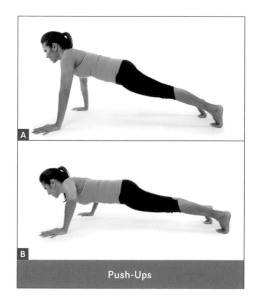

Push-Ups

Keep your chest open, with your shoulders back and down, away from your ears. Your head should be in line with your spine. Focus on the floor. Your entire body should feel solid, as if you're stuck in a tube.

GET MOVING: Bending your elbows and leading with your chest, lower your entire body to the floor and then straighten your arms to lift your entire body back up. Lower yourself as far as you can without sacrificing your form—even a mini push-up counts! Make sure you keep tipping your heels forward with every push-up. Maintain good posture and tap into your core strength for this workout.

SERIES: 20 pulses, *down/down*

LOOK OUT FOR: Keeping your hips too low or too high and arching or rounding your back as a result. Dropping your head. Rounding your shoulders and not squeezing your shoulder blades together on the way down. Placing your hands too close together or too far apart. Placing your hands too far forward and not in line with your shoulders. Arching your back instead of engaging your abs and tucking your hips slightly. Forgetting to tip your heels forward. Giving up because you can manage only a tiny range of movement.

NEED TO MODIFY? Tender wrists or tight shoulders: Make fists and substitute them for your flat palms. Tender back: Give yourself mini-breaks and be patient *or* do Push-Up Bent Knees (p. 88) instead.

TRANSITION: Lower your body straight down; flow into exercise 9.

9. Cobra

FOCUS: Core and back

BREATHING TECHNIQUE: Inhale your chest up/Exhale your hips forward and shoulders back.

GET IN POSITION: Begin by lying on your stomach, propped on your forearms. Slide your hands back under your shoulders, keeping your palms flat and fingertips spread. Keep your elbows bent, hugging them tightly into your body. Keep your feet and knees hip-width apart. Press the tops of your feet, thighs, and hips firmly into the floor.

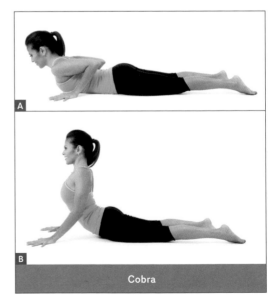

Cobra

Start to lengthen and straighten your arms while lifting your chest off the floor. Keep your shoulder blades back, puffing your ribs forward. Keep your hips connected to the floor and lift your upper body. (You might not be able to straighten your arms entirely, so feel free to keep your elbows slightly bent for comfort.) Firm up your butt and drive your hips forward while lifting your chest and stretching your abs. Twist your upper body to the right and to the left, lengthening your sides, and then return to center. (Repeat the movement twice.)

SERIES: 10-second hold

NEED TO MODIFY? Tender back: Do Cat/Cow (p. 99) instead.

TRANSITION: Come to your forearms; flow into exercise 10.

10. Forearm Plank Shift Series

FOCUS: Core and shoulders

INTENTION: "I will commit to the whole series; I'm getting stronger with each set."

GET IN POSITION: Begin by lying on your stomach, propped on your forearms. Your elbows should be in line with your shoulders. Keep your arms parallel, with your palms flat and fingertips spread. Keep your feet and thighs together. Clasp your hands together and interlace your fingers. Curl your toes under. By pressing into your forearms and toes, lift your entire body off the floor. Level and adjust your hips to be in line with your shoulders, creating a flat back. Keep your legs straight. Tighten your abs by pulling your belly button in toward your spine. Tuck your hips slightly so your back feels protected. Keep your chest open, with your shoulders back and down, away from your ears. Your head should be in line with your spine. Focus on the floor. Your entire body should feel solid, as if you're stuck in a tube.

GET MOVING: Continue to monitor the flatness of your body. Push away from the floor while maintaining good posture. Maintain straight legs. Keep your chest open and your head in line with your spine. Keep shifting your weight forward slightly. (Note: Move through the series swiftly; don't take too long of a break between sets!)

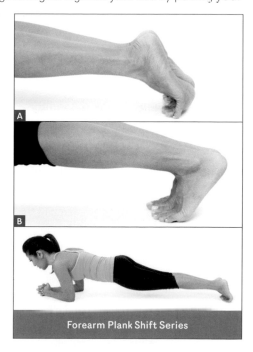

Forearm Plank Shift Series

SERIES: **Set 1:** *Hold* 1-minute hold Rest (a couple of seconds; not too long!) **Set 2:** *Shifts* 5-second hold 10 single count shifts *forward/backward* (Keep your back flat as you tip your heels and body forward and backward.) 10-second hold Rest (a couple of seconds; not too long!) **Set 3:** *Shifts/Pikes* 5-second hold 10 single count shifts *forward/backward* (same as earlier) 10 single count pikes *up/down* (Make a teepee with your body, shifting your weight out of your shoulders up toward ceiling, as in Down Dog.) 5-second hold Rest (a couple of seconds; not too long!)

LOOK OUT FOR: Keeping your hips too low or too high and arching or rounding your back as a result. Dropping your head. Rounding your shoulders. Sticking your butt up instead of engaging your abs and keeping a flat back. Arching your back instead of engaging your abs and tucking your hips slightly. Forgetting to maintain strong legs and pay attention to the sturdiness of your feet.

NEED TO MODIFY? Tender back: Give yourself mini-breaks and be patient *or* just do Plank (p. 63) instead.

TRANSITION: Slowly lower your body; flow into exercise 11.

11. Cobra

Repeat exercise 9.

TRANSITION: Come onto your hands and knees; flow into exercise 12.

12. Down Dog

Repeat exercise 4.

TRANSITION: Stay right there and lift your right leg; flow into exercise 13.

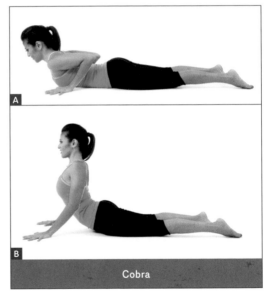

Cobra

13. One Leg Down Dog (Right)

FOCUS: Hamstrings and back

BREATHING TECHNIQUE: Inhale your arms long and hips and right leg up/ Exhale and ground your bottom left heel toward the floor.

GET IN POSITION: Begin in Down Dog. Extend your right leg up to the ceiling.

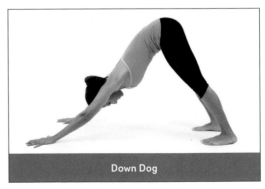

Down Dog

Keep your palms flat and fingers spread, parallel or slightly turned out. Open or square off your hips, whichever feels like a release. Start to lengthen your arms while lifting your right leg up higher. Push the top of your left thigh back and stretch your left heel down. Rotate your elbows in and firm up your arms and shoulders. Maintain a long back. Push away from the floor as your hips rise up and both legs get longer. Emphasize raising your left hip and opening your right hip. Keep your head in line with your arms; do not hang your head down.

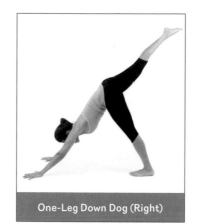

One-Leg Down Dog (Right)

SERIES: 10-second hold

NEED TO MODIFY? Tender knees or tight back and hamstrings: Keep your legs bent and heels raised.

TRANSITION: Step your right leg forward; flow into exercise 14.

14. Lunge (Right)

FOCUS: Thighs, glutes, and arms

INTENTION: "I'm pushing out doubt and building my strength."

GET IN POSITION: Begin with your feet hip-width apart, with your right foot about 2–3 feet in front of your left foot. Keep both of your feet parallel, with your toes in front of your heels. Raise your left heel off the floor. Bend both knees and drop your hips, forming a 90-degree angle with both legs. Tighten your abs by pulling your belly button in toward your spine. Lift your abs and chest up and away from your hips. Keep your chest open, with your shoulders back and down, away from your ears. Lift your arms up and across from your shoulders, forming a T-shape. Keep your palms facing down. Your head should be in line with your spine. Focus forward.

GET MOVING: Bend both of your knees as you lower your hips down and raise them up. Pretend your back is sliding up and down an imaginary wall, as you keep leaning your upper body back. Maintain a 90-degree angle with your right knee as you keep it in line with your right heel. Make sure your left heel is all the way up as you maintain a 90-degree angle with your left

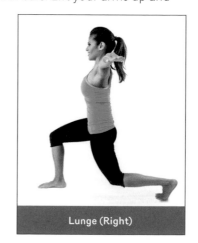

Lunge (Right)

knee. Keep reaching through your fingertips as you lengthen your arms and keep them up and across from your shoulders.

SERIES: 5-second hold 10 double count, *down/down/up/up* 10 single count, *down/up* 10 pulses, *down/down* 10-second hold

LOOK OUT FOR: Leaning forward and not maintaining a flat back. Bending your front knee too far over your front foot. Your back heel not being lifted high enough. Rounding your shoulders and chest. Not keeping your arms up and across from your shoulders.

NEED TO MODIFY? Tender knees: Keep your back leg straight and follow the same series.

TRANSITION: Lower your hands to the floor and step your right leg back; flow into exercise 15.

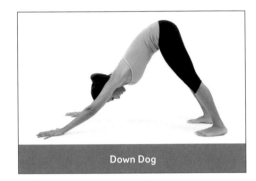
Down Dog

15. Down Dog

Repeat exercise 4.

TRANSITION: Walk your hands back on the floor; flow into exercise 16.

16. Ragdoll

FOCUS: Hamstrings

BREATHING TECHNIQUE: Inhale your hips up/Exhale your upper body toward the floor.

GET IN POSITION: Begin in Down Dog and walk your hands back toward your feet. Keep your feet parallel, with your toes in front of your heels. Grab hold of your elbows with your opposing hands. Maintain straight legs. (Soften your knees if your lower back or hamstrings are tight.) Keep folding your upper body over your legs, lengthening your spine. Hang, letting gravity pull your upper body toward the floor. Release any tension in your head and neck.

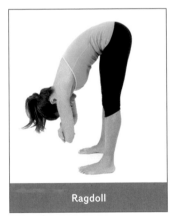
Ragdoll

SERIES: 10-second hold

NEED TO MODIFY? Tight hamstrings or back: Keep your legs bent. (Don't pressure yourself to straighten your legs.)

TRANSITION: Walk your hands forward on the floor; flow into exercise 17.

17. One Leg Down Dog (Left)

Repeat exercise 13, lifting your left leg.

TRANSITION: Step your left leg forward; flow into exercise 18.

18. Lunge (Left)

Repeat exercise 14 with your left leg forward.

TRANSITION: Lower your hands to the floor and step your right leg back; flow into exercise 19.

19. Down Dog

Repeat exercise 4.

TRANSITION: Walk your hands back on the floor; flow into exercise 20.

20. Ragdoll

Repeat exercise 16.

TRANSITION: Walk your hands forward on the floor; flow into exercise 21.

21. Plank Jumps

FOCUS: Core and shoulders

INTENTION: "Let me use control and not momentum to find my strength."

GET IN POSITION: Begin in Plank position with your hands in line with your shoulders, palms flat and fingertips spread. Keep your feet and thighs together. Straighten your legs. Tip your heels forward, as if you are stretching your feet and your body is about to take off. Level your hips and keep your back flat. Tighten your abs by pulling your belly button in toward your spine. Tuck your hips slightly so your back feels protected. Keep your chest open, with your shoulders back and down, away from your ears. Your head should

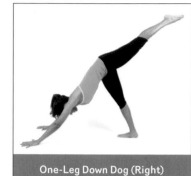

One-Leg Down Dog (Right)

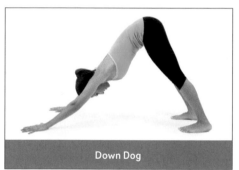

Lunge (Left)

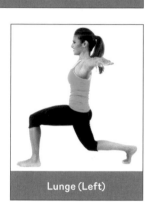

Down Dog

Ragdoll

be in line with your spine. Focus on the floor. Your entire body should feel solid, as if you're stuck in a tube.

GET MOVING: Continue to monitor the flatness of your body. Push away from the floor while maintaining good posture. Maintain straight legs. Keeping your hips level and back flat, jump your feet wider than your hips and then back together. Keep your chest open and your head in line with your spine. Keep shifting your weight forward slightly.

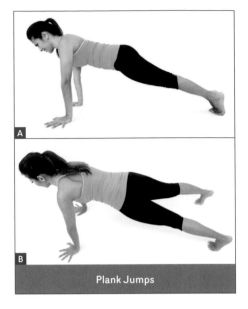

A

B

Plank Jumps

SERIES: 5-second hold 10 single count jump planks, *open/close* 10-second hold

LOOK OUT FOR: Keeping your hips too low or too high and arching or rounding your back as a result. Dropping your head. Rounding your shoulders. Placing your hands too close together or too far apart. Placing your hands too far forward and not in line with your shoulders. Bending your legs when jumping instead of keeping your legs straight. Arching your back instead of engaging your abs and tucking your hips slightly. Forgetting to tip your heels forward.

NEED TO MODIFY? Tender wrists or tight shoulders: Do Forearm Plank (p. 66) instead. Tender back: Give yourself mini-breaks and be patient *or* skip jumps and just hold Plank.

TRANSITION: Shift your weight and hips back and up; flow into exercise 22.

22. Down Dog

Repeat exercise 4.

TRANSITION: Walk your hands back and roll your body up; flow into exercise 23.

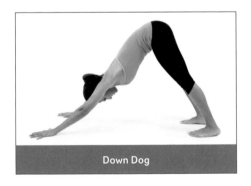

Down Dog

23. Standing Meditation

FOCUS: Total body awareness

MANTRA: No one can take away your happiness.

BREATHING TECHNIQUE: Inhale your chest up/Exhale your shoulders back.

GET IN POSITION: Begin by standing with your feet hip-width apart. Keep your feet parallel, with your toes in front of your heels. Maintain straight legs. Point your tailbone down. Tighten your abs by pulling your belly button in toward your spine. Stand tall as you lengthen your abs and chest up and away from your hips. Keep your chest open, with your shoulders back and down, away from your ears. Your head should be in line with your spine. Focus forward. Bring your palms together in front of your chest.

SERIES: 30-second hold or longer

NEED TO MODIFY? Close your eyes to help you focus better.

TRANSITION: Stay standing; flow into exercise 24.

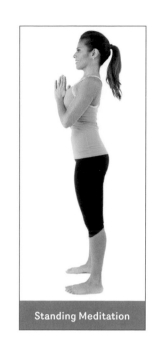

Standing Meditation

24. Standing Leg Lifts (Right)

FOCUS: Thighs

INTENTION: "Let me stand tall and proud and achieve balance."

GET IN POSITION: Begin by standing with your feet in a V-shape (heels together, toes apart). Lift your arms up and across from your shoulders, forming a T-shape. Keep your palms facing down. Slightly bend both knees, keeping them in line with your toes. Extend your right leg out in front of your body, flexing your right foot (heel into the floor) and turning your toes up to the ceiling. Engage your right thigh and lift your leg an inch off the floor, keeping your foot flexed. Point your tailbone down. Tighten your abs by pulling your belly button in toward your spine. Lift your abs and chest up and away from your hips. Keep your chest open, with your shoulders back and down, away from your ears. Keep your head in line with your spine. Focus forward.

GET MOVING: Ground your left foot into the floor and lift your right leg up as high as possible without involving your hip. Move your leg for the whole series without touching the floor, keeping your leg as straight

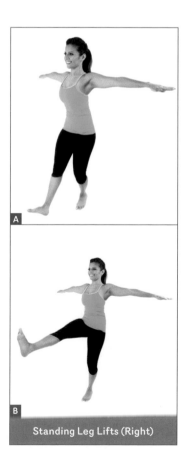

Standing Leg Lifts (Right)

DOUBT

as possible. Isolate your thigh. (Imagine a box sitting on top of your thigh that is being lifted up and down.) Maintain your posture and tap into your core strength.

SERIES: 10 double count, *up/up/down/down*, full range (right foot almost to the floor and then up and in front of your hip) 10 single count, *up/down*, full range (right foot almost to the floor and then up and in front of your hip) 10 pulses, *up/up* (Foot stays at hip level.) 10-second hold (at hip level)

LOOK OUT FOR: Leaning too far back as a result of lifting your leg too high or not being aware of your posture. Not maintaining level hips. Swinging your leg instead of making deliberate movements. Touching your heel to the floor. Using your hip flexor instead of your thigh muscle to lift your leg.

NEED TO MODIFY? Feeling your hip flexor instead of your thigh: Bend your knee slightly and play around with the rotation of your leg. Tight back: Hold onto the wall for support.

TRANSITION: Step your right leg back; flow into exercise 25.

25. Warrior 1 (Left)

FOCUS: Hips and thighs

BREATHING TECHNIQUE: Inhale and reach your arms up and press your right heel down/ Exhale and bend your left knee forward and drop your left thigh lower.

GET IN POSITION: Begin in lunge position with your left foot about 2–3 feet in front of your right foot. Keep your left foot parallel, with your toes in front of your heels. Turn your right foot out at a 45 or 60-degree angle, keeping your foot flat on the floor. Try to align your heels. Square your hips by turning your right hip forward and pulling your left hip back. Raise your arms straight up to the ceiling. Keep your palms facing in and reach strongly through your fingertips. Bend your left knee at a 90-degree angle over your left ankle. Try to get your left thigh parallel to the floor. In order to align properly, feel free to adjust your left foot forward or back accordingly. Tighten your abs by pulling your belly button in toward your spine. Lift your abs and chest up and away from your hips. Keep your chest open, with your shoulders back and down, away from your ears. Continue to reach your arms up toward the ceiling. Focus forward. (Or, you can tilt back slightly and look up at your thumbs.)

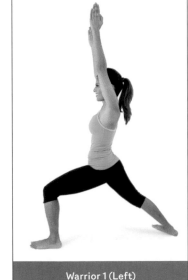

Warrior 1 (Left)

SERIES: 5 breaths, *inhale/exhale* Make sure to take long, full breaths.

NEED TO MODIFY? Tender knees or tight back and hamstrings: Keep your back heel raised slightly *or* shorten the space between your legs.

TRANSITION: Lower your arms and turn to the right; flow into exercise 26.

26. Warrior 2 (Left)

FOCUS: Hips and thighs

BREATHING TECHNIQUE: Inhale and lift your chest up and reach your arms out to the sides/Exhale and bend your left knee forward, drop your left thigh lower, and ground your right heel.

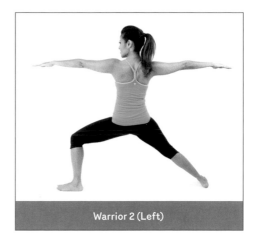

Warrior 2 (Left)

GET IN POSITION: Begin in Warrior 1 position. Turn your right foot out at a 90-degree angle, keeping your foot flat on the floor. Try to align your heels. Square your hips by pulling your right hip back and your left hip forward. (Keep them as wide open as possible.) Raise your arms straight across from your shoulders into a T-shape. Keep your palms facing down and reach strongly through your fingertips. Bend your left knee at a 90-degree angle over your left ankle. Try to get your left thigh parallel to the floor. In order to align properly, feel free to adjust your left foot forward or backward accordingly. Tighten your abs by pulling your belly button in toward your spine. Lift your abs and chest up and away from your hips. Keep your chest open, with your shoulders back and down, away from your ears. Keep your shoulders in line with your hips. (Be careful not to lean forward.) Continue to reach your arms away from one another. Turn your head to the left and focus forward in line with your left arm.

SERIES: 5 breaths, *inhale/exhale* Make sure to take long, full breaths.

NEED TO MODIFY? Tender knees or tight back and hamstrings: Keep your back heel raised slightly *or* shorten the space between your legs.

TRANSITION: Turn and step your right leg forward to stand; flow into exercise 27.

27. Standing Leg Lifts (Left)

Repeat exercise 24, lifting your left leg.

TRANSITION: Step your left leg back; flow into
exercise 28.

28. Warrior 1 (Right)

Repeat exercise 25 on your right side.

TRANSITION: Lower your arms and turn to the left; flow
into exercise 29.

29. Warrior 2 (Right)

Repeat exercise 26 on your right side.

TRANSITION: Turn and step your left leg forward to
stand; flow into exercise 30.

30. Standing Meditation

Repeat exercise 27. Repeat the mantra.

MANTRA: No one can take away your happiness.

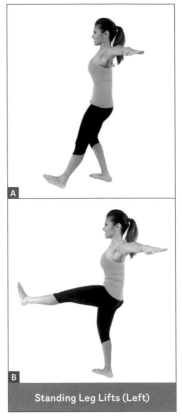

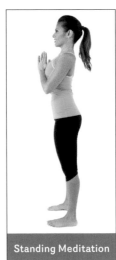

Standing Leg Lifts (Left)

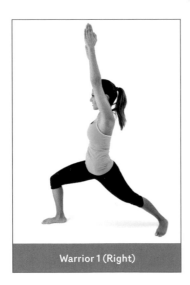

Warrior 1 (Right)

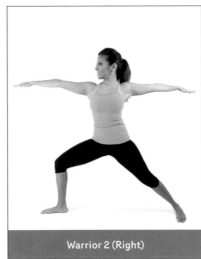

Warrior 2 (Right)

Standing Meditation

THE POST-WORKOUT

1 **Post-Workout Recap:**

Be proud of yourself. You took your doubt and fears, pushed past them, and encouraged yourself to successfully accomplish a well-deserved goal.

Did my emotional weight change?

☐ YES   ☐ NO

Did I accomplish my workout intention?

☐ YES   ☐ NO

Is there a change in my physical body?

☐ YES   ☐ NO

2 **My Post-Workout Mood Is:**

(Write down, think, or say out loud.)

_____

DOUBT

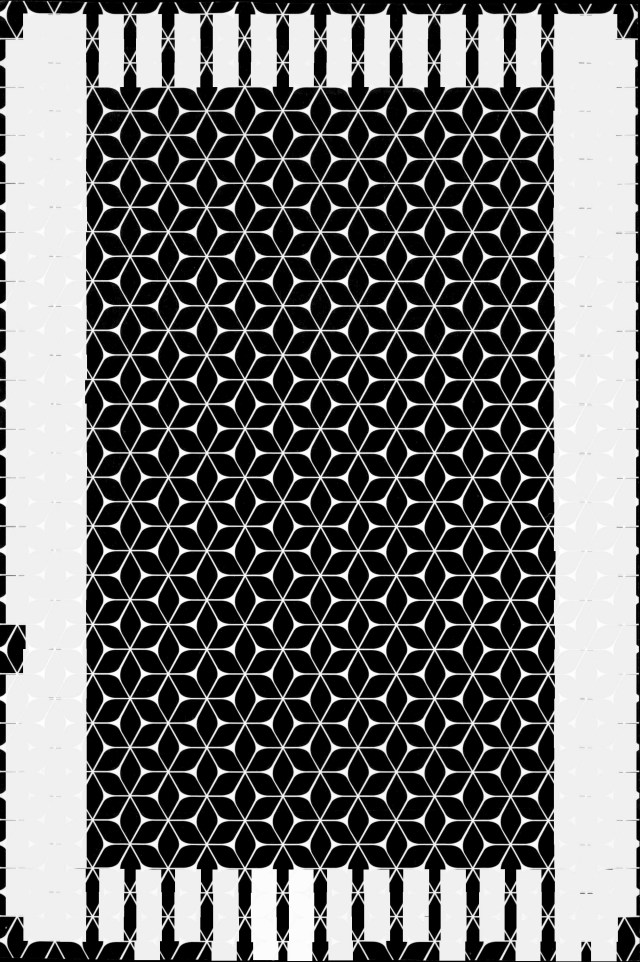

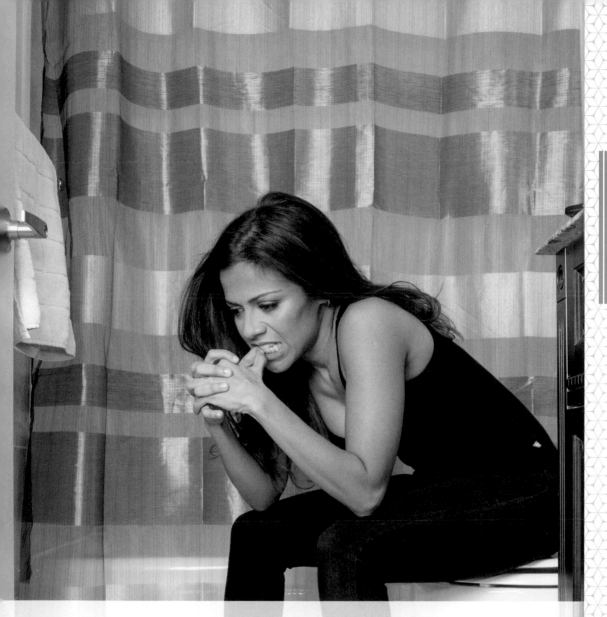

— CHAPTER 9 —

THE ANXIETY WORKOUT

THE ANXIETY EXERCISES

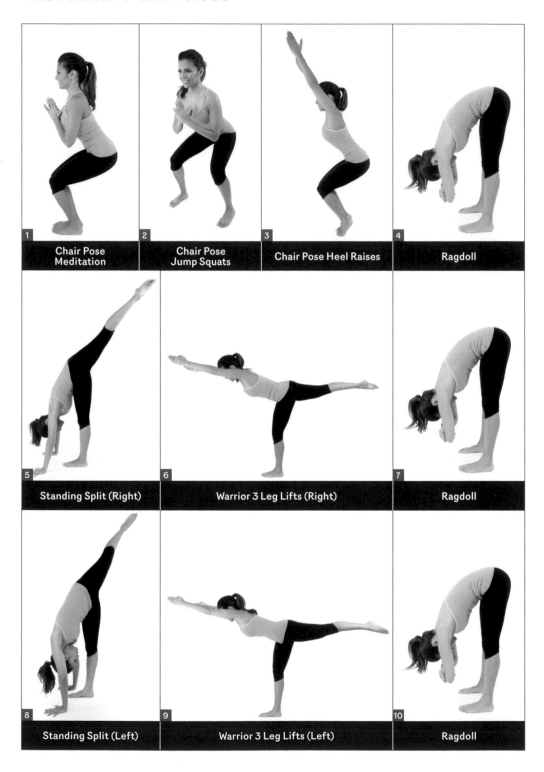

1. Chair Pose Meditation
2. Chair Pose Jump Squats
3. Chair Pose Heel Raises
4. Ragdoll
5. Standing Split (Right)
6. Warrior 3 Leg Lifts (Right)
7. Ragdoll
8. Standing Split (Left)
9. Warrior 3 Leg Lifts (Left)
10. Ragdoll

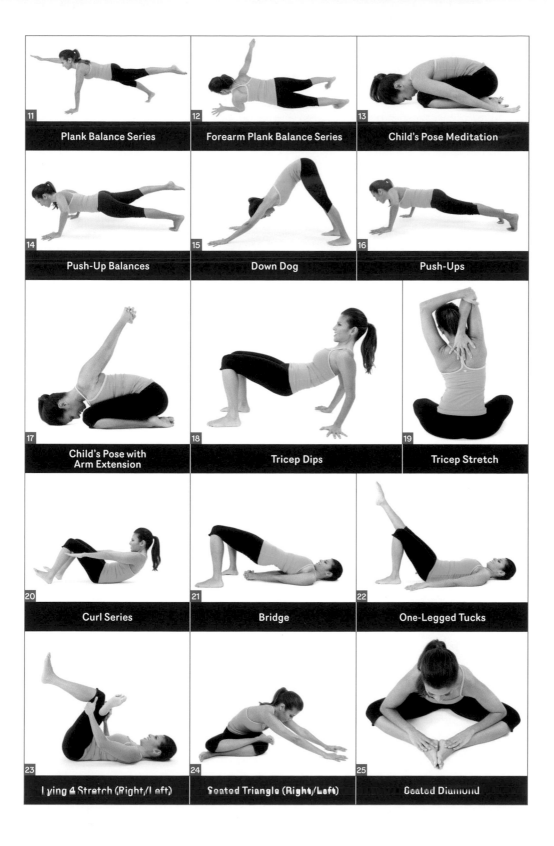

11 Plank Balance Series

12 Forearm Plank Balance Series

13 Child's Pose Meditation

14 Push-Up Balances

15 Down Dog

16 Push-Ups

17 Child's Pose with Arm Extension

18 Tricep Dips

19 Tricep Stretch

20 Curl Series

21 Bridge

22 One-Legged Tucks

23 Lying 4 Stretch (Right/Left)

24 Seated Triangle (Right/Left)

25 Seated Diamond

Anxiety can be overwhelming—and much longer-lasting than regular stress. It is often discounted and misunderstood, and can be rooted in acute and deep fears that seem impossible to overcome. It is an emotion that can gnaw at you so incessantly you feel as if you are being eaten alive. The road of anxiety can leave you lost as you strive for a conclusion, a game plan, anything to stop the feeling. With no destination in sight, you can end up feeling helpless—so it's no wonder you feel paralyzed. You're simultaneously starring in and watching a scary movie. It's all too much and all-encompassing.

Ask yourself this: What is that one anxious thought you keep coming back to? The thought that makes you feel worried all over? The thought that is making you feel so fearful you feel you need a team of experts working around the clock to annihilate it from your mind? That is the thought I want you to own.

What is the emotional weight of that thought and its resulting mood, and how is it manifesting in your physical body?

THE PRE-WORKOUT

1 **I Am Feeling:**

☐ Agitated	☐ Doubtful	☐ Perturbed
☐ Angst	☐ Fearful	☐ Preoccupied
☐ Anxious	☐ Fretful	☐ Qualms
☐ Apprehensive	☐ Frustrated	☐ Shaky
☐ Bothered	☐ Fussy	☐ Tense
☐ Careworn	☐ Gloomy	☐ Touchy
☐ Concerned	☐ Harried	☐ Troubled
☐ Crippled	☐ High-Strung	☐ Uncomfortable
☐ Depressed	☐ Isolated	☐ Uneasy
☐ Despondent	☐ Misgivings	☐ Unnerved
☐ Desultory	☐ Nerve-Wracked	☐ Upset
☐ Detached	☐ Nervous	☐ Vexed
☐ Disquieted	☐ Overwhelmed	☐ Wary
☐ Distressed	☐ Panicked	☐ Worried

Choose from the list above, or add your own words. Then write down your mood *or* say it out loud and embrace it.

2 My Current Mood Is:

_____

3 My Emotional Weight Is:

1   5   10

Light   Neutral   Heavy

4 My Physical Symptoms Are:

☐ Acid Reflux	☐ Heartburn	☐ Rapid Breathing
☐ Adrenaline Rush	☐ Heavy Breathing	☐ Rapid Heartbeat
☐ Chills	☐ Heavy Chest	☐ Shaking
☐ Cramps	☐ Jaw Clenching	☐ Stomachache
☐ Crying	☐ Jittery	☐ Sweating
☐ Dizziness	☐ Nausea	☐ Teeth Grinding
☐ Goosebumps	☐ Neurosis	☐ Tightness
☐ Hand-Wringing	☐ Pacing	☐ Tingling
☐ Headaches	☐ Panic Attacks	

TEN COMMON ANXIOUS THOUGHTS

- I'm going to be late and miss that plane and I'll never get where I'm going.
- This headache won't go away. What if it never goes away? What if I have a brain tumor?
- How am I going to get pregnant? We've been trying for so long and I'm getting old.
- Will I die in the plane/car/train/bus/subway?
- I think my new boss hates me. Please, oh please, don't let me get fired.
- Are they going to find out that I lied?
- How will I be able to pay my rent this month?
- I'm not worried about the holidays. I'm just anxious about being worried.
- What will happen if we get divorced?
- I'll never be good enough to get the job done the way I want it.

THE WORKOUT

1 Mantra for Anxiety:

Don't magnify success or failure.

The word *anxiety* makes me anxious! And that's how simple the anxiety process can be: starting with one tiny word. Flying, career, health, cancer, secrets, marriage, bills—hear or say any of these words, and all of a sudden you could be taking a fast trip to Anxious Town in your head.

I've found that when I'm experiencing life through the lens of anxiety, everything is heightened and magnified . . . and not in a good way. One momentary failure can suddenly equal a failed *life*: I didn't fail just one test, I've been bad at tests since I was born and I'll never pass another one. One success plus a quick ego can get me attached to future anxieties: A simple scenario of me getting married can quickly morph into thoughts like, "When are we going to have kids and how can we afford them and what if I have problems with my pregnancy and what if our baby gets sick" . . . See what I mean? What ifs are killer. Anxiety is king in the realm of the hypothetical.

To magnify something is an intentional act that requires tools. Our tools—our bodies, minds, and hearts—are what we use to see and experience the world. Magnifying our successes or failures makes them bigger than they are—we use our minds and hearts to do this. And this is where anxiety comes into play.

Even though we are often taught to regard success and failure as opposites, when we magnify them and get attached to the outcome, they can both bring equally destructive emotions. You could feel pressure to succeed or fail; you could feel entitled to a congratulations or to sympathy; you could feel that you will never fail or that you will never succeed and be surprisingly unprepared for both. More than anything, you could feel anxious because of your attachment to both real and hypothetical outcomes.

If you tend to fall into the pattern of magnifying your successes and failures, you could be setting yourself up for chronic anxiety. Instead, by choosing *not* to magnify them, you can be liberated from that burden. And with that freedom comes the ability to accurately evaluate, actively appreciate, and genuinely accept all moments in life— the successes *and* the failures. Through this acceptance, you level the playing field and become more grounded, as you allow yourself to win at the game of life.

I learned this, not surprisingly, from my dad, who always seems to have the last word. If I think a conversation is over and done, it's *not*! He typically ends a conversation by sharing an old saying, a story from his childhood (usually one I've heard a million times), or a repeated point. Being on the receiving end of constant feedback has felt comforting, challenging, and annoying. I can call my dad after feeling like I failed and am guaranteed a powerful vote of support and a realistic evaluation. He will automatically put out the fire of my anxieties, so whatever situation I'm dealing with seems much more manageable. I can also call my dad after feeling like I succeeded and be met with uninvited, yet always loving, feedback and constructive criticism. My dad's unsolicited support, advice, and persistent push to reflect make me feel the important impact of his mantra: "Don't magnify success or failure."

This mantra is challenging because it requires finding the delicate balance between achievements and disappointments. During times of failure, this lesson is incredibly comforting. During times of success, it is deeply humbling. During times of anxiety, it is deeply calming, and lets the butterflies in my stomach fly away.

No matter how much success or failure I experience in my life, my dad has a unique way of making me see both my successes and failures as nothing more than fleeting moments. He waves a magic wand of soothing words, "Don't magnify success or failure," and my anxiety diminishes in an instant. The weight is taken away—and we know how important *that* is!

My father strongly believes that if we choose to magnify these things, we get attached to the successes and failures of others and ourselves, seeing them as fixed definitions of our true character and overall achievement. We disregard feelings of humility, forgiveness, love, sharing, and teaching—the requirements for growth that truly define our humanity.

In fact, magnifying successes and failures not only stunts our growth but also isolates us and deepens our worries, attaching us to increased feelings of entitlement, pressure, and insecurity. Anxiety will prevent you from being fully in the moment and able to realistically assess what's going on.

It's easy to give examples of huge successes and failures that can bring about anxiety, like getting the job of your dreams or getting divorced. The "Don't magnify success or failure" mantra actually comes down to the power of *smaller* moments. Little stressors can lead to big anxieties.

When I was in third grade, my teacher called my parents to tell them that I was not only disruptive in class but that math was extremely difficult for me. She was personally discouraged and not hopeful about my progress. I was frantic. I couldn't sleep. I was a failure at math already and thought it meant I probably would not have a bright future. And the worst part was, I couldn't charm my way out of it. No matter how nice I was, everyone was about to discover how dumb and unteachable I really was. That anxiety ate me alive and I was only eight years old!

My father could have chosen to magnify this and to get mad at me for not trying hard enough or for misbehaving, but he didn't. He sat down with me and said that when he has trouble learning things, sometimes all he needs is a different approach. He helped me photocopy each page of my math book and said I could even make a new cover for the book and call it whatever I wanted. We went through my new book every night. Without pressure, my dad reassured me that all he expected was for me to try, to tell him when I didn't understand something, and to trust him. I did, and after six months math became my favorite subject. Instead of magnifying what my teacher saw as a failure, he merely saw it as a moment, helped me in an encouraging and loving way, and we moved on. My anxiety melted away, and I've had a love for numbers ever since.

Another third-grade experience comes to mind in support of this mantra. I loved dancing and wanted to be a ballerina. I was the star at the end-of-year performance at my ballet school. I received many compliments and was so proud of myself. I asked my dad repeatedly if I was the best. He told me he was proud of me and wanted to know each detail of my experience and how I felt. The next day, my family and I watched my dad's video of the performance. I could see on his face how proud he was of me but also how happy he was for the other dancers. He chose not to magnify my success. He forced me to focus on the experience rather than the outcome. As a result, I felt closer to the other girls, and our performance became a bonding moment instead of one ripe with potential anxieties, which soon could have sprouted into "Will I be the best next year? What should I do next if I sprain my ankle? What if a new girl comes into school and is better than I? What if we get a new teacher?"

Without this lesson, small successes and failures can turn into larger issues, bringing in unbalanced egos, uncompromising viewpoints, misinterpreted securities, and even more anxiety. My dad believes that the "Don't magnify success or failure" mantra greatly contributes to his healthy marriage of over fifty years to my mom. My dad and mom can come home and say to each other, "I messed up," yet know that they have each other's support no matter what. They also know that if they come home with successes, they will be met with excitement and loving space to potentially fail. This freedom helps reduce the heaviness of anxiety and maintain a delicate balance of happiness in my home.

My dad's purpose in sharing this lesson was not to dim the light of success or ignore the sting of failure, but rather to encourage an autonomy that exists when you are unattached to outcomes. His grounded approach to life is what I strive to remember whenever my anxieties pop up and threaten to overwhelm me. I think of his wise words and stop viewing my worries through a huge magnifying glass.

Instead of using the power of success and failure to conjure up what ifs and anxieties, see them as equal in what they can offer us. That way, you'll be able to calm yourself as you discover and relish the unmagnified and accurate foundation of a resolve that can exist in both success and failure for all of us.

2 **How to Use the Mantra**

When you're really anxious, all you can do is focus on the situation that you fear could spiral out of control, right? Can you mold your heightened anxiety into a place where the worries can be flat-lined and then neutralized?

Strive to take all that adrenaline and use it to reshape your tower of fear into a field of calm. Focus on that nervous feeling in the pit of your stomach and let your concentration move it to a place where the nerves slowly but surely evaporate. Remember, anxiety is the great magnifier. It always makes things seem or feel worse than they are. Knowing you have the power to find perspective and demagnify this anxiety should take a huge weight off your shoulders.

Convert your anxiety diet of fear and panic to focus and perspective. Repeat the "Don't magnify success or failure" mantra as much as you need to and commit to a balanced and focused workout.

3 **Why the Anxiety Workout**

By now you have taken the time to reflect on the source of your anxiety and how it weighs on you emotionally and physically.

The flow of this exercise series is designed for you to keep in constant motion to distract you from your worrisome mood. You will be challenged with elements of concentration and coordination, doing a lot of balance work to keep you focused on anything other than your state of mind. This will ultimately leave you feeling energized yet calmer and more centered.

Embrace your mood, reflect on the mantra, and let it provide you with the perspective needed to find acceptance in a challenging routine based upon a delicate balance of coordination and stillness.

4 **My Anxiety Workout Intention (Emotional or Physical) Is:**
(Write down, think, or say out loud.)

5 The Anxiety Exercises

1. Chair Pose Meditation

FOCUS: Thighs, back, and glutes

MANTRA: Don't magnify success or failure.

BREATHING TECHNIQUE: Inhale your arms up/Exhale your hips down. Embrace a sense of perspective.

GET IN POSITION: Begin by standing with your feet and knees together. Keep your feet parallel, with your toes in front of your heels. Keep your knees in line with your heels as you bend your knees and drop your hips, trying to get your thighs parallel to the floor. Press your feet firmly into the floor. Lean forward slightly with your upper body until your back and thighs form a 90-degree angle. Keep your back flat as you

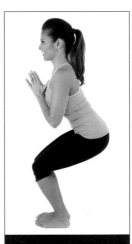

Chair Pose Meditation

bring your palms together in front of your chest. Tighten your abs by pulling your belly button in toward your spine. Keep your shoulders back and down, away from your ears. Keep pressing your palms together firmly. Keep your tailbone down. Put more pressure on your heels, shifting your weight back. Your head should be in line with your spine. Focus forward.

SERIES: 5 breaths, *inhale/exhale*

NEED TO MODIFY? Tender knees or back: Keep your hips up higher.

TRANSITION: Stay focused and jump right into exercise 2.

2. Chair Pose Jump Squats

FOCUS: Thighs and glutes

INTENTION: "Let me find my steadiness, my core."

GET IN POSITION: Begin by standing in Chair Pose with your feet and knees together. Keep your feet parallel, with your toes in front of your heels. Keep your knees in line with your heels as you bend your knees and drop your hips, trying to get your thighs parallel to the floor. Press your feet firmly into the floor. Lean forward slightly with your upper body until your back and thighs form a 90-degree angle. Keep your back flat as you bring your palms together in front of your chest. Tighten your abs by pulling your belly button in toward your spine. Keep your shoulders back and down, away from your ears. Keep pressing your palms together firmly. Keep your tailbone down. Put more pressure on your heels, shifting your weight back. Your head should be in line with your spine. Focus forward.

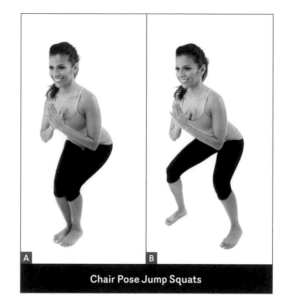

Chair Pose Jump Squats

GET MOVING: Keep your core steady and palms together as you jump your bent legs out to the sides into a wide squat (think wide-legged chair pose). Jump back and forth between a wide-legged chair pose and a regular chair pose, keeping your upper body steady. Throughout the movement, maintain the chair pose angle in your body. Keep your abs engaged and your core steady. Try to stay at the same height/angle with each jump out/in. Make sure your toes stay in line with the direction of your knees.

SERIES: 20 single count, *out/in* (Jump out and in.)

LOOK OUT FOR: Being too bouncy and not tapping into the steadiness and strength of your jump. Leaning forward and sticking your butt out. Bad posture. Jumping unevenly. (Put the same effort into each leg.) Turning your feet out instead of keeping them parallel.

NEED TO MODIFY? Tender knees: Stay up higher *or* skip jumping and step out and in instead.

TRANSITION: Stay in chair pose; flow into exercise 3.

3. Chair Pose Heel Raises

FOCUS: Thighs, back, and glutes

INTENTION: "Let me enjoy my pure strength."

GET IN POSITION: Begin by standing in Chair Pose with your feet and knees together. Keep your feet parallel, with your toes in front of your heels. Keep your knees in line with your heels as you bend your knees and drop your hips, trying to get your thighs parallel to the floor. Press your feet firmly into the floor. Lean forward slightly with your upper body until your back and thighs form a 90-degree angle. Keep your back flat and extend your arms straight up to the ceiling. Tighten your abs by pulling your belly button in toward your spine. Your arms should be parallel to your shoulders with your shoulders back and down, away from your ears. Face your palms toward one another and reach through your fingertips. Keep your tailbone down. Put more pressure on your heels, shifting your weight back. Your head should be in line with your spine. Focus forward.

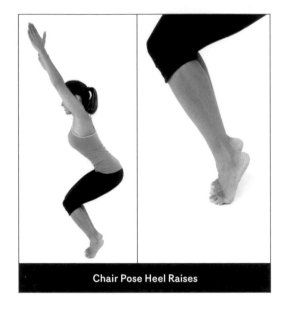

Chair Pose Heel Raises

GET MOVING: Raise your heels all the way up and hold, then lower back down to flat feet. Balance on the balls of your feet while maintaining chair pose. A good trick is to keep your eyes focused on the same point and level the whole series. Keep your abs engaged and your core steady. Breathe and find power in your feet. Isolate the sensation in your thighs.

SERIES: 5-second hold, *feet flat* 10-second hold, *heels raised* 5-second hold, *feet flat* 10-second hold, *heels raised* 5-second hold, *feet flat* 10-second hold, *heels raised* 10-second hold, *feet flat*

LOOK OUT FOR: Not raising your heels high enough. Gripping with your toes instead of pressing them firmly and evenly into the floor. Leaning forward and sticking your butt out. Bad posture. Sinking your hips too low and bending your knees too much.

NEED TO MODIFY? Tender knees: Stay up higher *or* raise your toes up and down for only one interval.

TRANSITION: Fold your body over and walk your feet wider; flow into exercise 4.

4. Ragdoll

FOCUS: Hamstrings

BREATHING TECHNIQUE: Inhale your hips up/Exhale your upper body toward the floor.

GET IN POSITION: Begin by standing with your feet hip-width apart. Keep your feet parallel, with your toes in front of your heels. Reach your arms toward the floor as you fold your upper body over your legs, lengthening your spine. Grab hold of your elbows with your opposing hands. Maintain straight legs. (Soften your knees if your lower back or hamstrings are tight.) Hang, letting gravity pull your upper body toward the floor. Release any tension in your head and neck.

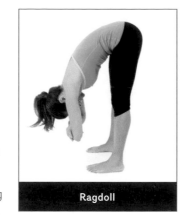

Ragdoll

SERIES: 10-second hold

NEED TO MODIFY? Tight hamstrings or back: Keep your legs bent. (Don't pressure yourself to straighten your legs.)

TRANSITION: Place your hands on the floor and lift your right leg; flow into exercise 5.

5. Standing Split (Right)

FOCUS: Hamstrings

BREATHING TECHNIQUE: Inhale and reach your right leg up/Exhale and draw your chest toward your left thigh.

GET IN POSITION: Begin by standing in a forward bend with your hands on the floor. Play around with the placement of your hands (closer in/farther away), depending on your comfort and flexibility. Shift your weight onto your left foot and slowly extend your right leg up toward the ceiling. Try to straighten both legs. Bring your chest in toward your left leg. Keep your left leg parallel to your right, with your knee facing forward. Avoid rolling to the outer edge of your left foot by pressing on the inner edge of your left foot. Keep your right leg straight, toes pointed. Open or square off your hips, whichever feels like a release. Play around with keeping your right leg parallel or turned out; do what feels good. Maintain a connection to both legs and don't get caught up in how

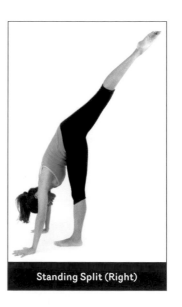

Standing Split (Right)

high your right leg is. Maintain a long back. Engage your abs and draw your chest and hands closer to your left leg. Emphasize raising your right leg and grounding your left leg. Keep your head in line with your arms. You should feel balanced on your left foot.

SERIES: 10-second hold

NEED TO MODIFY? Tight hamstrings: Keep your legs slightly bent and don't walk your hands in as much.

TRANSITION: Lift your arms and lower your right leg; flow into exercise 6.

6. Warrior 3 Leg Lifts (Right)

FOCUS: Hamstrings, glutes, back, and arms

INTENTION: "Balancing only gets better when you practice balancing. I have to commit."

GET IN POSITION: Begin by standing with your feet hip-width apart. Keep your feet parallel, with your toes in front of your heels. Keep your left foot flat and leg sturdy as you extend your right leg behind you. Lean forward and raise your right leg up to be in line with your hip. Keep your right leg parallel to the left with your knee facing the floor and your foot flexed. Square your hips by turning your right hip down. Square your shoulders by turning your right shoulder down. You can place your hands on your hips to help align your hips and shoulders. Try to establish a flat back with your shoulders in line with your hips. Lengthen both legs without locking your bottom knee. Tighten your abs by pulling your belly button in toward your spine. Extend your arms straight forward in line with your shoulders, palms facing in. Keep your chest open, with your shoulders back and down, away from your ears. Keep your head in line with your spine. You should feel long as you stretch your head forward and your right heel back. Focus forward.

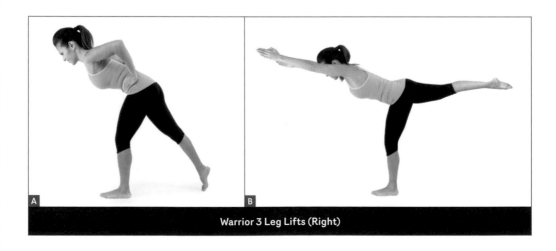

Warrior 3 Leg Lifts (Right)

GET MOVING: Ground your left foot into the floor and lower and lift your right leg. Move your leg for the whole series without touching the floor, keeping your leg as straight as possible. Isolate your butt. (Imagine a box sitting on top of your butt that you're trying to keep balanced.) Keep your body long, stretching your arms away from your right leg. Maintain your posture and tap into your core strength.

SERIES: 20 single count, *down/up*, full range (right foot almost to the floor and then up and across from your hip) 20 pulses, *up/up* (Foot stays at hip level.) 5-second hold (at hip level)

LOOK OUT FOR: Not maintaining level hips. Collapsing your head and shoulders. Arching your back. Swinging your leg instead of making deliberate movements. Touching your foot to the floor. Not bringing your leg high enough and across from your hip. Getting frustrated, stopping and starting too easily. (Try to balance!)

NEED TO MODIFY? Tender ankle: Use a wall for support and slowly train yourself to balance. Tender back: Don't bring your right leg up as high.

TRANSITION: Lower your right leg and upper body; flow into exercise 7.

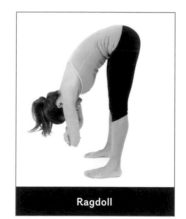

Ragdoll

7. Ragdoll

Repeat exercise 4.

TRANSITION: Place your hands on the floor and lift your left leg; flow into exercise 8.

8. Standing Split (Left)

Repeat exercise 5 on your left side.

TRANSITION: Lift your arms and lower your left leg; flow into exercise 9.

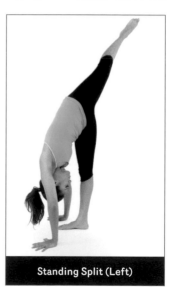

Standing Split (Left)

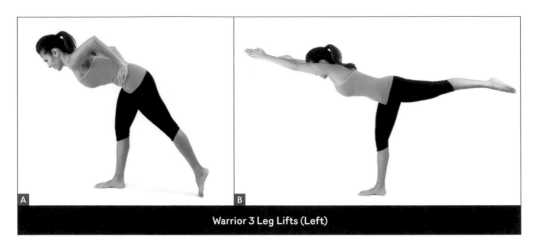

Warrior 3 Leg Lifts (Left)

9. Warrior 3 Leg Lifts (Left)

Repeat exercise 6 on your left side.

TRANSITION: Lower your left leg and upper body; flow into exercise 10.

10. Ragdoll

Repeat exercise 4.

TRANSITION: Walk your hands forward on the floor; flow into exercise 11.

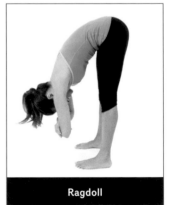

Ragdoll

11. Plank Balance Series

FOCUS: Core and shoulders

INTENTION: "Practice makes perfect, and this gets better with practice."

GET IN POSITION: Begin in Plank position with your hands underneath your shoulders, palms flat and fingertips spread. Keep your feet hip-width apart. Straighten your legs. Tip your heels forward, as if you are stretching your feet and your body is about to take off. Level your hips and keep your back flat. Tighten your abs by pulling your belly button in toward your spine. Tuck your hips slightly so your back feels protected. Keep your chest open, with your shoulders back and down, away from your ears. Your head should be in line with your spine. Focus on the floor. Your entire body should feel solid, as if you're stuck in a tube.

GET MOVING: Continue to monitor the flatness of your body. Push away from the floor while maintaining good posture. Maintain straight legs. Try the whole balance series while maintaining steadiness, alignment, and form. Keep your chest open and your head in line with your spine. Keep shifting your weight forward slightly. (Note: Don't get frustrated; stop and start if need be—balancing is hard!)

SERIES: 10-second hold 10-second hold, right leg (Lift up only your right leg.) 10-second hold, left leg (Lift up only your left leg.) 10-second hold, right arm (Lift up only your right arm.) 10-second hold, left arm (Lift up only your left arm.) 10-second hold, right leg/left arm (Lift up both your right leg and left arm.) 10-second hold, left leg/right arm (Lift up both your left leg and right arm.) 10-second hold (original plank position)

LOOK OUT FOR: Keeping your hips too low or too high and arching or rounding your back as a result. Dropping your head. Rounding your shoulders. Placing your hands too close together or too far apart. Placing your hands too far forward and not in line with your shoulders. Giving up easily because balancing feels wobbly. Arching your back instead of engaging your abs and tucking your hips slightly. Forgetting to tip your heels forward.

NEED TO MODIFY? Tender wrists or tight shoulders: Do Forearm Plank (p. 66) instead or skip balancing. Tender back: Give yourself mini-breaks and be patient.

TRANSITION: Come to your hands and knees and take a quick breather; flow into exercise 12.

12. Forearm Plank Balance Series

FOCUS: Core and shoulders

INTENTION: "My concentration will help me get balanced."

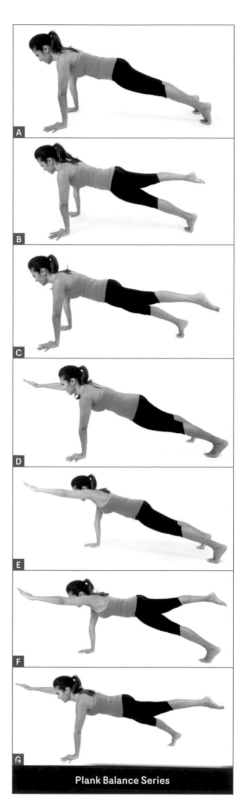

Plank Balance Series

ANXIETY

GET IN POSITION: Begin by lying on your stomach, propped on your forearms. Your elbows should be in line with your shoulders. Keep your arms parallel, with your palms flat and fingertips spread. Keep your feet hip-width apart. Curl your toes under. By pressing into your forearms and toes, lift your entire body off the floor. Level and adjust your hips to be in line with your shoulders, creating a flat back. Keep your legs straight. Tighten your abs by pulling your belly button in toward your spine. Tuck your hips slightly so your back feels protected. Keep your chest open, with your shoulders back and down, away from your ears. Your head should be in line with your spine. Focus on the floor. Your entire body should feel solid, as if you're stuck in a tube.

GET MOVING: Continue to monitor the flatness of your body. Push away from the floor while maintaining good posture. Maintain straight legs. Try the whole balance series while maintaining steadiness, alignment, and form. Keep your chest open and your head in line with your spine. Keep shifting your weight forward slightly. (Note: Don't get frustrated; stop and start if need be—balancing is hard!)

SERIES: 10-second hold 10-second hold, right leg (Lift up only your right leg.) 10-second hold, left leg (Lift up only your left leg.) 10-second hold, right arm (Lift up only your right arm.) 10-second hold, left arm (Lift up only your left arm.) 10-second hold, right leg/left arm (Lift up both your right leg and left arm.) 10-second hold, left leg/right arm (Lift up both your left leg and right arm.) 10-second hold (original forearm plank position)

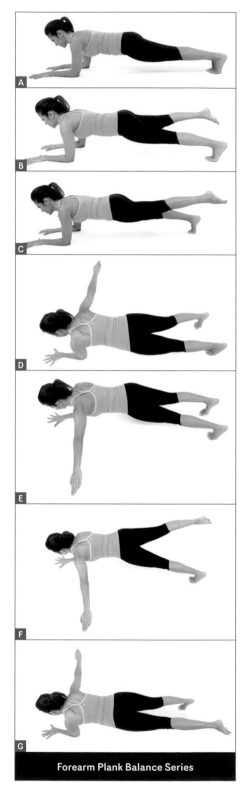

Forearm Plank Balance Series

LOOK OUT FOR: Keeping your hips too low or too high and arching or rounding your back as a result. Dropping your head. Rounding your shoulders. Sticking your butt up instead of engaging your abs and keeping a flat back. Giving up easily because balancing feels wobbly. Arching your back instead of engaging your abs and tucking your hips slightly. Forgetting to maintain strong legs.

NEED TO MODIFY? Tender wrists or tight shoulders: Do Plank (p. 63) instead *or* skip balancing. Tender back: Give yourself mini-breaks and be patient.

TRANSITION: Shift your weight and rest back; flow into exercise 13.

13. Child's Pose Meditation

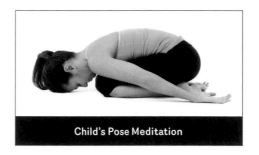

Child's Pose Meditation

FOCUS: Shoulders and back

MANTRA: Don't magnify success or failure.

BREATHING TECHNIQUE: Inhale and exhale; observe your chest rising and falling. Embrace a sense of calm.

GET IN POSITION: Begin by kneeling on the floor and sitting on your heels. Your feet should be comfortably together, with your knees apart and wider than your hips. Fold your upper body forward between your thighs and bring your forehead to the floor. Place your straight arms back alongside your torso with your palms up. Release your shoulders toward the floor.

SERIES: 10-second hold

NEED TO MODIFY? Tender knees: Place a pillow under your hamstrings for elevation *or* play around with the placement of your knees until you feel comfortable.

TRANSITION: Shift your weight forward into your hands; flow into exercise 14.

14. Push-Up Balances

FOCUS: Chest, arms, and core

INTENTION: "Even if it is tiny, it counts—and I'm getting stronger."

GET IN POSITION: Begin in Plank position with your hands wider than your shoulders, palms flat and fingertips spread. Keep your feet hip-width apart. Straighten your legs. Tip your heels forward, as if you are stretching your feet and your body is about to take off. Level your hips and keep your back flat. Tighten your abs by pulling your belly button in toward your spine. Tuck your hips slightly so your back feels protected. Keep your chest open, with your shoulders back and down, away from your ears. Your head should be in line with your spine. Focus on the floor. Your entire body should feel solid, as if you're stuck in a tube.

GET MOVING: Raise your right leg up and bring your right foot up in line with your right hip. Point your toes. Keep your right leg up and do a push-up by bending your elbows, lowering your entire body to the floor, and then straightening your arms to lift your entire body back up. Lower yourself as far as you can without sacrificing your form—even a mini push-up counts! Make sure you keep tipping your left heel forward with every push-up. Maintain good posture and tap into your core strength for this workout. Repeat the movement on your left side.

SERIES: 10 single count, *down/up* (Lift up only your right leg.) 10 single count, *down/up* (Lift up only your left leg.) 10 pulses, *down/down* (original push-up position both feet down)

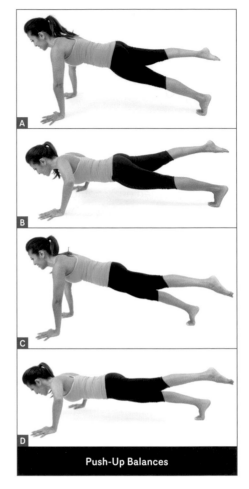

Push-Up Balances

LOOK OUT FOR: Keeping your hips too low or too high and arching or rounding your back as a result. Dropping your head. Rounding your shoulders and not squeezing your shoulder blades together on the way down. Placing your hands too close together or too far apart. Placing your hands too far forward and not in line with your shoulders. Not lifting your top leg high enough and aligning your foot in line with your hip. Arching your back instead of engaging your abs and tucking your hips slightly. Forgetting to tip your heels forward. Giving up because you can manage only a tiny range of movement.

NEED TO MODIFY? Tender wrists and tight shoulders: Make fists and substitute them for your flat palms. Tender back: Give yourself mini-breaks and be patient *or* do Push-Up Bent Knees (p. 88) instead.

TRANSITION: Shift your weight and hips back and up; flow into exercise 15.

15. Down Dog

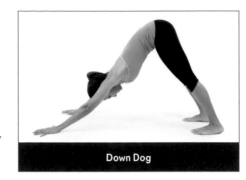

Down Dog

FOCUS: Hamstrings and back

BREATHING TECHNIQUE: Inhale your arms
long and hips up/Exhale your shoulders
down and heels toward the floor.

GET IN POSITION: Beginning in Plank position,
make sure your hands are slightly in front
of your shoulders. Your palms (parallel or
slightly turned out) should be flat and your fingers spread. Keep your toes curled as you
shift your weight back and lift your hips up toward the ceiling. As you start to lengthen
your arms and legs, continue to press your palms and heels down. As your hips rise
toward the ceiling, push the tops of your thighs back and stretch your heels down to
the floor, lengthening your hamstrings. Straighten your knees but do not lock them.
Maintain straight legs. (Soften your knees if your lower back or hamstrings are tight.)
Rotate your elbows in to firm up the arms and shoulders. Maintain a long back. Keep
your head in line with your arms; do not hang your head down. (Note: Imagine you're
creating a teepee with your body!)

SERIES: 10-second hold

NEED TO MODIFY? Tender knees or tight back and hamstrings: Keep your legs bent and
heels raised.

TRANSITION: Shift your weight forward and place your hands wider; flow into exercise 16.

16. Push-Ups

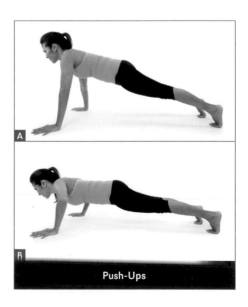

Push-Ups

FOCUS: Chest, arms, and core

INTENTION: "Even if it is tiny, it counts—and
I'm getting stronger."

GET IN POSITION: Begin in Plank position
with your hands wider than your shoulders,
palms flat and fingertips spread. Keep your
feet hip-width apart. Straighten your legs.
Tip your heels forward, as if you are stretching your feet and your body is about to take
off. Level your hips and keep your back flat.
Tighten your abs by pulling your belly button
in toward your spine. Tuck your hips slightly

so your back feels protected. Keep your chest open, with your shoulders back and down, away from your ears. Your head should be in line with your spine. Focus on the floor. Your entire body should feel solid, as if you're stuck in a tube.

GET MOVING: Bending your elbows and leading with your chest, lower your entire body to the floor and then straighten your arms to lift your entire body back up. Lower yourself as far as you can without sacrificing your form—even a mini push-up counts! Make sure you keep tipping your heels forward with every push-up. Maintain good posture and tap into your core strength for this workout.

SERIES: 20 pulses, *down/down*

LOOK OUT FOR: Keeping your hips too low or too high and arching or rounding your back as a result. Dropping your head. Rounding your shoulders and not squeezing your shoulder blades together on the way down. Placing your hands too close together or too far apart. Placing your hands too far forward and not in line with your shoulders. Arching your back instead of engaging your abs and tucking your hips slightly. Forgetting to tip your heels forward. Giving up because you can manage only a tiny range of movement.

NEED TO MODIFY? Tender wrists or tight shoulders: Make fists and substitute them for your flat palms. Tender back: Give yourself mini-breaks and be patient *or* do Push-Up Bent Knees (p. 88) instead.

TRANSITION: Shift your weight and rest back; flow into exercise 17.

17. Child's Pose with Arm Extension

FOCUS: Shoulders and chest

BREATHING TECHNIQUE: Inhale your arms up and forward toward your head/Exhale your lower back and hips down.

GET IN POSITION: Begin by kneeling on the floor and sitting on your heels. Your feet should be comfortably together, with your knees apart and wider than your hips. Fold your upper body forward between your thighs and bring your forehead to the floor. Clasp your hands together behind your back and reach your arms straight up toward the ceiling and forward toward your head. Rock your arms from side to side.

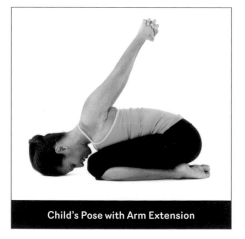

Child's Pose with Arm Extension

SERIES: 10-second hold

NEED TO MODIFY? Tender knees: Place a pillow under your hamstrings for elevation *or* play around with the placement of your knees until you feel comfortable.

TRANSITION: Roll your body up and bring your legs out in front of you, flow into exercise 18.

18. Tricep Dips

FOCUS: Triceps

INTENTION: "Let me train myself to feel the targeted triceps and not give up."

GET IN POSITION: Begin by sitting on the floor with your hands placed comfortably behind your back. Bend your knees at a 90-degree angle, keeping your feet flat on the floor. Your hands should be placed under your shoulders, hugging your hips in. Turn your palms out at a 90-degree angle. Keep your palms flat and spread your fingertips. Lean back and press into your feet and hands to lift your hips up from the floor. Balance on your hands and feet as you straighten your arms and press your hips up to be level with your knees and shoulders. Shift your body back into your hands again, aligning your shoulders slightly behind your wrists.

GET MOVING: Bend your elbows down toward the floor and toward one another and then straighten your arms to lift back up. Try to keep your hips up and the rest of your body steady as you bend and drop your elbows only. Zero in on and isolate just your triceps to do the work.

SERIES: 10 single count, *down/up* 10 pulses, *down/down* 10 single count, *down/up*

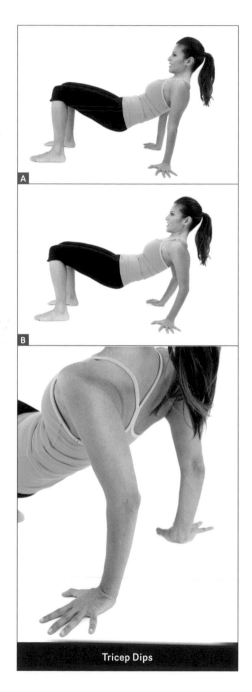

Tricep Dips

LOOK OUT FOR: Dropping your hips instead of just your elbows. Not leaning back into your hands. Letting your elbows bend out to the sides instead of in toward one another. Misplacing your palms, either not turning them out enough or turning them in too much.

NEED TO MODIFY? Tender wrists: Stay seated and bend your elbows (skip lifting your hips up). Tight shoulders: Place your hands wider apart.

TRANSITION: Sit on the floor; flow into exercise 19.

19. Tricep Stretch

FOCUS: Triceps

BREATHING TECHNIQUE: Inhale your chest and elbow up/Exhale your shoulder down. Inhale and lean back/Exhale and lean to the side.

GET IN POSITION: Begin in a cross-legged seated position. Extend your right arm straight up toward the ceiling, keeping your hand in line with your shoulder. Bend your right elbow, and place your right palm behind you onto your right shoulder blade. Place your left hand on top of your right elbow. Use your left hand to pull your right arm up higher as you start to lift your upper body up. Lean back as you lengthen your abs and chest up and away from your hips. Keep your chest open, with your shoulders back and down, away from your ears. Continue to lift your right elbow as you push

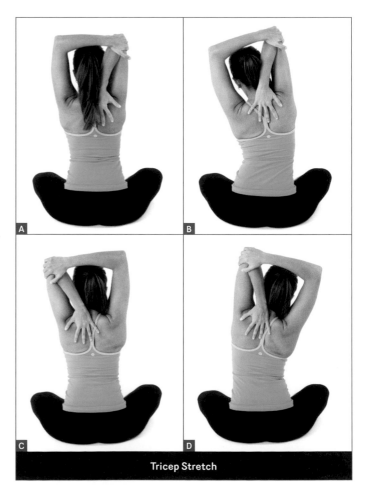

Tricep Stretch

your shoulders down. Lean slightly to the left for an added release. Your head should be in line with your spine. Focus forward. Repeat the movement on your left side.

SERIES: 10-second hold, right side 10-second hold, left side

NEED TO MODIFY? Tight shoulders: Take your opposite hand to your upper arm instead of your elbow.

TRANSITION: Rest back onto your forearms; flow into exercise 20.

20. Curl Series

FOCUS: Core

INTENTION: "This is supposed to be tough. I want things challenging and effective. I'm going to let go of any ego; I will strive for proper form as opposed to feeling pressure to be too advanced."

GET IN POSITION: Begin by lying flat on your back. Bend your knees and draw your feet toward your butt, forming a 90-degree angle with your knees. Keep your feet and knees hip-width apart and parallel. (Feel free to play around with your foot placement, closer together or wider apart, to get comfortable.) Keep your feet flat on the floor, with your toes in front of your heels. Prop yourself up on your forearms. Your elbows should be in line with your shoulders. Keep your arms parallel, with your palms flat and fingertips spread. Your abs should be pulling down and back and your chest should be curling over your abs. Keep your shoulders down. Engage your abs by pulling them in tightly and scooping your hips up. (Create a letter "C" with your body.) Your core should feel solid (as if you're wearing a tight seatbelt). (Note: Tackle the form here and be patient. Your attention to your core and feet can make all the difference.) Press your lower back into the floor. Keep your head in line with your spine. Focus forward.

GET MOVING: From your forearms, observe your eye level and make sure it is in line with your knees. Maintain that eye level while grabbing your outer thighs with your hands. Keep your elbows wide and your shoulders down as you hollow out your upper body. Create a deeper "C" with your back by pulling your belly button toward your spine, grounding your lower back, and pulling your shoulders down. Your chest should curl over your abs. (Imagine your chest "eating" your abs.) Keep all movements small. (Don't read into a small range of motion.) When curling, it should feel as if you hit a wall with each curl: that "wall" is you pulling your abs tight. Let go of your thighs only if you're ready! When you let go, your feet will flex, with your heels digging into the floor to help ground and stabilize. If your upper body drops too much when you let go, it's not worth it!

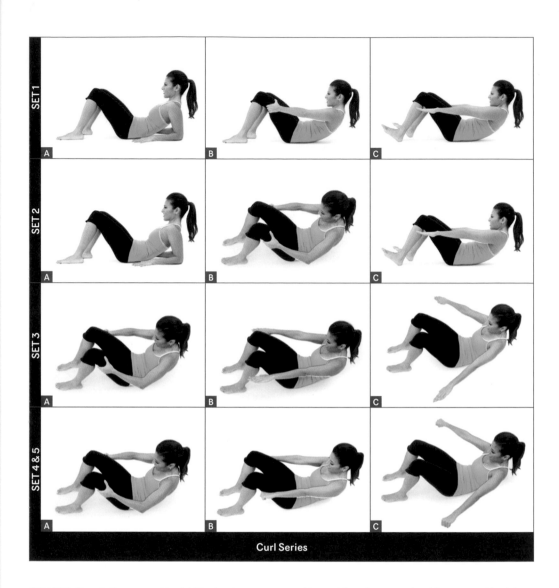

Curl Series

SERIES: **Set 1**: 5-second hold 10 single count, *up/down* 10 pulses, *up/up* 10-second hold release (Release your arms to your sides and flex your feet.)* Rest on your forearms (a couple of seconds, not too long!) **Set 2**: 5-second hold 10 single count, *up/down* 10 pulses, *up/up* 10 single count release, *up/down* (release your arms to your sides and flex your feet)* Rest on your forearms (a couple of seconds, not too long!) **Set 3**: 5-second hold 10 single count, *up/down* 10 pulses, *up/up* 10 single count release taps, *out/in* (Release your arms to your sides and tap in and away from your knees.)* Rest on your forearms (a couple of seconds, not too long!) **Set 4**: 5-second hold 10 single count, *up/down* 10 pulses, *up/up* 10 single count release combo, *out/in/up/down* (Release your arms to your sides, make fists and tap out and into your knees and then curl up and down.)* Rest on your forearms (a couple of seconds, not too long!) **Set 5:** 5-second hold 10 single count release combo, *out/in/up/down* (Release your arms to your sides, make fists and tap out and into your knees and then curl up and down.)* 10-second hold release (Hold the last curl and keep your arms released.)*

*Don't feel pressure to let go. Master holding on as that is what builds your strength most effectively. If letting go makes you feel unstable and/or lose form, it's not worth it. Do the same series while holding on and try to ground your feet.

LOOK OUT FOR: Rounding your shoulders too much. Staying too low and using your neck to pull forward. Not maintaining eye level with your knees. Not using your arms enough or using them too much. Using your back instead of your abs to lift your upper body. Not grounding your feet. Being too ambitious with releasing your arms. Forgetting to breathe!

NEED TO MODIFY? Weak abs: Continue to hold on *or* let go of one arm at a time and alternate. Back or hip issues: Come up higher or go down lower in your curl. Tightness in neck or shoulders: Put a towel under your legs and hold onto the towel instead of your thighs.

TRANSITION: Lie back on floor; flow into exercise 21.

21. Bridge

FOCUS: Back and glutes

BREATHING TECHNIQUE: Inhale your chest up/Exhale and ground your heels and push your hips up.

GET IN POSITION: Begin by lying flat on your back with your legs bent at a 90-degree angle and your feet flat on the floor. Keep your feet and knees hip-width apart and parallel. Keep your toes in front of your heels. Your arms should be straight down by your sides with your palms up. Gently push your hips and back up off the floor. Clasp your hands and interlace your fingers under your butt. Push your hips up higher until your thighs are parallel to the floor. As you push your hips up, shimmy your shoulders under you as you extend through your arms. Push your chest toward your face and roll your shoulders down and toward one another.

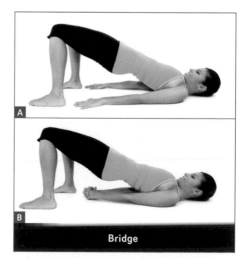

Bridge

Keep your knees in line with your heels. Feel your knees pull away from your hips as you lengthen your tailbone toward the backs of your knees.

SERIES: 20-second hold

NEED TO MODIFY? Tight back: Don't lift too high *or* Do Cat/Cow instead.

TRANSITION: Stay on the floor; flow into exercise 22.

22. One-Legged Tucks

FOCUS: Glutes, hips, and inner thighs

INTENTION: "I can have fun right now."

GET IN POSITION: Begin by lying flat on your back. Bend your knees and draw your feet toward your butt, keeping your feet flat on the floor. Keep your feet hip-width apart. (Feel free to play around with your foot placement, closer together or wider apart, to get comfortable.) Keep your toes in front of your heels. Keep your right knee steady as you lift your right shin and extend your right toes out in front of you. Engage your right thigh as you point your toes. Keep your thighs parallel, with your knees across from one another. Repeat the movement on your left side.

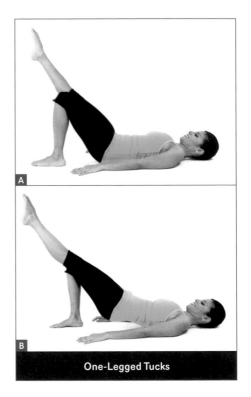

One-Legged Tucks

GET MOVING: Engage your abs by pulling them in tightly and pressing your back into the floor. Tucking your pelvis under, move just your butt up and down off the floor. (Try to find a good beat with your butt lifts, like you're bouncing a basketball.) Maintain a small range of motion. (Less is more!) Make sure to keep your abs engaged and your back flat as you isolate your butt to lift your hips. You're flipping your hips up toward your chest, doing a mini-lift with your butt. Keep in mind that you will feel more of a strain on the side that is grounded (the foot on the floor).

SERIES: 20 single count, *up/down*, (Right leg up.) 20 multi-count, *up/up/up/down*, (Right leg up.) 5-second hold, (Right leg up.) 20 single count, *up/down*, (Left leg up.) 20 multi-count, *up/up/up/down*, (Left leg up.) 5-second hold, (Left leg up.)

LOOK OUT FOR: Using your whole back to lift just your butt up. (Your back should not be off the floor.) Swinging your hips too high off the floor. Placing your feet too close to your butt. (Be nice to your knees!) Bringing your top leg too high and not keeping your thighs parallel.

NEED TO MODIFY? Tender knees: Walk your feet in closer *or* flex your feet.

TRANSITION: Stay on the floor; flow into exercise 23.

23. Lying 4 Stretch (Right/Left)

FOCUS: Glutes

BREATHING TECHNIQUE: Inhale your left knee into your chest/Exhale your right knee away from your chest as you lower your back to the floor. Inhale your right knee into your chest/Exhale your left knee away from your chest as you lower your back to the floor.

GET IN POSITION: Begin by lying flat on your back with your legs bent at a 90-degree angle and your feet flat on the floor. Lift your right leg up and gently place your right ankle on top of your left thigh, close to your left knee. Flex your right foot. Lift your left foot off the floor as you draw your knees and legs in toward your chest. Flex your left foot. Thread your arms through your legs, interlacing your fingers behind your left leg. Use your right elbow (or hand) to help you press and turn your right knee and thigh away from your body as you draw your left knee and thigh in toward your body. Press your butt down toward the floor while continuing to draw your left knee in. Repeat the movement on your left side.

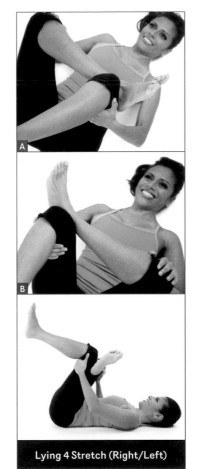

Lying 4 Stretch (Right/Left)

SERIES: 10-second hold, right side (right ankle to left thigh) 10-second hold, left side (left ankle to right thigh)

NEED TO MODIFY? Tight hips or back: Keep the foot of your bottom leg on the floor instead of lifting it toward your chest.

TRANSITION: Roll forward to sit up; flow into exercise 24.

24. Seated Triangle (Right/Left)

FOCUS: Glutes and hips

BREATHING TECHNIQUE: Inhale as you reach your arms to the left/Exhale as you pull your right hip back and down. Inhale as you reach your arms to the right/Exhale as you pull your left hip back and down.

GET IN POSITION: Begin in a cross-legged seated position. Using your hands, gently place your right ankle on top of your left knee, aligning your right shin with your left shin. Flex your right foot. Adjust your left foot so that it is in line with your right knee (thus creating a "triangle" between your thighs). Don't worry if there is a lot of space between your right knee and your left foot and you don't "look" flexible; the feet and knees being aligned is more important. Place your palms on the floor by your sides. Using your hands to help you, reach your hips back as you fold your upper body forward. Draw your chest toward your shins. Walk both of your arms to your left side, in line with your right foot. Continue to reach and walk your fingertips and arms out to the left as you resist and press your right hip down toward the floor. Repeat the movement on your left side.

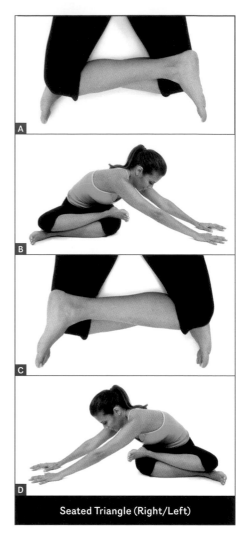

Seated Triangle (Right/Left)

SERIES: 10-second hold, right side (right leg on top, arms to your left) 10-second hold, left side (left leg on top, arms to your right)

NEED TO MODIFY? Tight hips: Do Lying T-Stretch (p. 60) instead.

TRANSITION: Sit up and uncross your feet; flow into exercise 25.

25. Seated Diamond

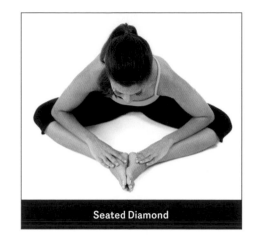

Seated Diamond

FOCUS: Hips, groin, and back

MANTRA: Don't magnify success or failure.

BREATHING TECHNIQUE: Inhale your chest forward/Exhale your hips back. Inhale your chest forward/Exhale your knees apart. Embrace your commitment.

GET IN POSITION: Begin in a seated position. Create a diamond shape with your legs by placing the soles of your feet together in front of your groin. Move your feet closer in or farther away from you to find your "sweet spot." Place your elbows or your hands into the creases of your knees. Using your elbows or hands, press your knees apart. Press your chest forward as you pull your hips back.

SERIES: 10-second hold

NEED TO MODIFY? Tight hips or back: Place your feet farther away from your body.

THE POST-WORKOUT

1 Post-Workout Recap:

Be proud of yourself. You took your anxiety and channeled those nerve-wracking worries into a productive and grounding workout.

Did my emotional weight change?

☐ YES   ☐ NO

Did I accomplish my workout intention?

☐ YES   ☐ NO

Is there a change in my physical body?

☐ YES   ☐ NO

2 My Post-Workout Mood Is:

(Write down, think, or say out loud.)

PART III
MOOD FOOD

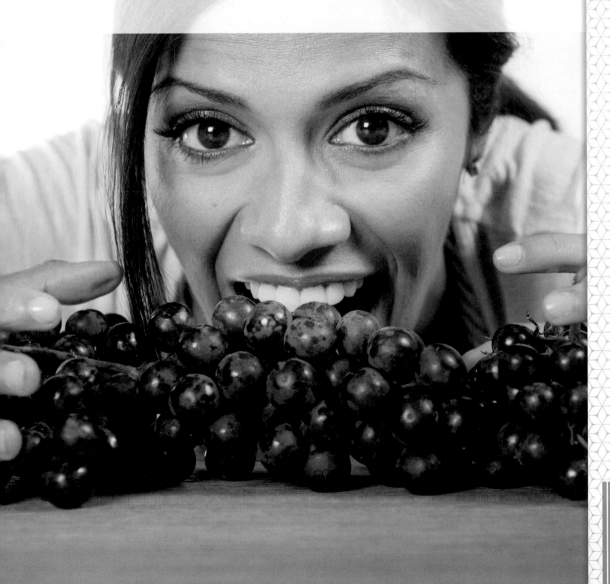

— CHAPTER 10 —
MOOD-FOOD BASICS

I've never been a strict dieter and I love all kinds of foods. In fact, when I'm following a rigid diet, I tend to be more anxious and out of my natural balance. I find I'm my healthiest when I'm eating what feels right for me. Rather than following diets that force me to change my entire grocery list, I am drawn to simple, practical changes that make immediate differences.

A little can go a long way. A simple and healthy vitamin, herb, or new smoothie recipe can often make me feel better. For example, when I was told I should drink a glass of water first thing in the morning, it changed my life more than any diet could have. It encouraged me to slow down the first few minutes of my day. Eventually that grew into making time for better, healthier breakfasts. Sometimes it takes just one suggestion to open the door to your healthy mood-food journey.

Given this mindset, I decided to tap into one of the world's oldest holistic systems, Ayurveda, a Sanskrit word that means "science of life." I used this to devise a simple plan to help you choose foods that can make a tremendous difference, depending on your mood and your body.

According to Ayurvedic science, all living creatures and their environments are composed of five basic elements: Fire, Air, Earth, Water, and Space. The predominance of these elements falls into three categories, or *doshas*: Vata, Pitta, and Kapha. Each person is a unique combination of these elements and their doshas. I'm a Vata/Pitta mix.

The food philosophy of Ayurveda is based on the composition and qualities of foods that best create nourishment for your dosha and lead to satisfaction, healthy emotions, clear thoughts, and contentment in mind and soul. Based on your dosha, combining foods that are compatible with each other, as well as combining them with harmonious spices and herbs, can help balance and stabilize your moods and physical health. As everyone has a specific constitution and unique state of balance, Ayurveda prescribes maintaining this balance of elements through food as a way to establish or maintain health, as having an imbalance may lead to disease.

Ayurveda also describes six tastes of food: sweet, sour, salty, pungent, bitter, and astringent. By knowing your dosha, you can single out the specific tastes you need to increase or decrease throughout the day to have a positive effect on your disposition.

I consulted Dr. Aparna Bapat, an accredited Ayurvedic expert, and Roxy Naba, a skilled chef, from the Hamptons and New York City (whose meals always put me in a good mood!). We created several lists to help you easily figure out your dosha, optimal mood-food snacks, as well as six unique mood mixers to jump-start a better mind and body. As you know, life happens and moods change, so mix up your mood mixers!

DOSHA: Vata

IF YOU ARE VATA, YOU TEND TO BE:

Physically

- Small-boned
- Lean and tall, may have difficulty gaining weight
- Likes to stay active

Emotionally

- Lively and enthusiastic
- Has a short attention span
- Has difficulty making decisions
- Prone to anxiety
- Hyperactive

HOW VATA RESPONDS TO THE SEVEN MOODS	
■ Anger	Erratic and sudden outbursts that blow over quickly
■ Energy	Impulsive bursts, then tires easily
■ Stress	Feels constricted and overwhelmed
■ Chill	Very blissful and calm
■ Happiness	Expresses with joy and physical movement like dancing or singing
■ Doubt	Deep insecurity and not knowing what to say or do
■ Anxiety	Restless thoughts, mindless actions (nail biting, teeth grinding)

DOSHA: Pitta

IF YOU ARE PITTA, YOU TEND TO BE:

Physically

- Medium-boned
- Gains weight evenly
- Likes competitive physical activities

Emotionally

- Outgoing and assertive
- Logical, rational thinker
- Enjoys planning and organizing
- Talkative
- Prone to passionate outbursts

HOW PITTA RESPONDS TO THE SEVEN MOODS	
■ Anger	Intense fury, may hold a grudge
■ Energy	Sustained, driven, and focused
■ Stress	Feels a competitive need to prove oneself while suppressing true emotions
■ Chill	Very hard to relax; occurs usually when there is nothing left to gain from fighting the feeling
■ Happiness	Often comes from achievements and sharing them
■ Doubt	Obsessed with details to confidently justify doubt to self and others
■ Anxiety	Scattered thoughts, self-harm (scratching, lip biting)

DOSHA: Kapha

IF YOU ARE KAPHA, YOU TEND TO BE:

Physically

- Heavy-boned
- Gains weight easily, especially in the lower body
- Prefers not to work out

Emotionally

- Easygoing and friendly
- A cautious thinker
- Prefers a regular routine
- Sentimental
- Understanding

HOW KAPHA RESPONDS TO THE SEVEN MOODS	
■ Anger	Rarely lasts long, mostly internalized, passive-aggressive
■ Energy	Patient, enduring
■ Stress	Needs to be in control
■ Chill	A normal state of mind
■ Happiness	Genuine goodwill and cheerful smile
■ Doubt	Self-reassurance that things really aren't so bad
■ Anxiety	Repetitive thoughts and actions (holding head in hands, gazing down)

Food Choices and Best Antidotes for Your Dosha

VATA

A Vata constitution is the combination of Air and Space. Foods that are similarly dry, light, cold, or rough can increase these same qualities. When a Vata person consumes such food in excess they can become slender, quick, anxious, active, imaginative, bloated, dehydrated, constipated, or restless. Moderate consumption will help them to maintain balance.

Go-to Foods

Sesame oil; warm cooked food (denser whole grains and root vegetables like barley and carrot stew); ginger tea; rice and wheat; cooked vegetables like beets, carrots, and asparagus; chicken, turkey, seafood, and eggs.

Mood-Food Snack Suggestions

- oatmeal
- orange juice
- bananas
- cantaloupe
- rice or rice pudding
- dates
- avocado dip (guacamole)
- roasted nuts
- hard-boiled eggs

PITTA

A Pitta constitution is the combination of Fire and Water. Foods that are spicy, sour, or acidic maintain Pitta balance when consumed in moderation. In excess, they create imbalances like acidity, burning, stress, anger, bleeding, and hormonal imbalances.

Go-to Foods

Ghee (clarified butter); cooling cardamom milk (milk steeped with whole cardamom); coconut; cucumbers, broccoli, cauliflower, asparagus, beets, and dark leafy greens; coriander seeds; chicken, turkey, and pheasant; alkaline foods, rice, barley, and oats.

Mood-Food Snack Suggestions

- granola
- dried sweet fruits like raisins
- almond milk
- pumpkin or sunflower seeds
- pomegranates
- mangos
- grapes
- apples
- figs
- cherries

KAPHA

A Kapha constitution is the combination of Earth and Water. Foods that are sweet, starchy, greasy, dense, congestive, and stale can increase Kapha qualities if consumed in excess. This can create weight gain, fatigue, mucus, accumulation of fluid, or blockages. With portion and quality control, the right foods can help maintain a healthy balance.

Go-to Foods:

Honey; garlic; black pepper; gluten-free foods (like quinoa); roasted vegetables with pungent spices and lemon; beans (minus soybean); tomatoes, zucchini, asparagus, and green beans; barley and buckwheat; chicken breast, turkey, eggs, and seafood.

Mood-Food Snack Suggestions

- plain popcorn
- cereal
- celery
- berries
- apricots
- peaches
- pears
- salt-free crackers
- radishes

TASTE CHOICES FOR YOUR DOSHAS WHEN YOU'RE OUT OF BALANCE

IF YOU ARE VATA

Increase:	Sweet, Sour, and Salty
Decrease:	Astringent, Bitter, and Pungent

IF YOU ARE PITTA

Increase:	Bitter, Sweet, and Astringent
Decrease:	Pungent (spicy and oily), Salty, and Sour

IF YOU ARE KAPHA

Increase:	Pungent, Astringent, and Bitter
Decrease:	Sweet, Salty, and Sour

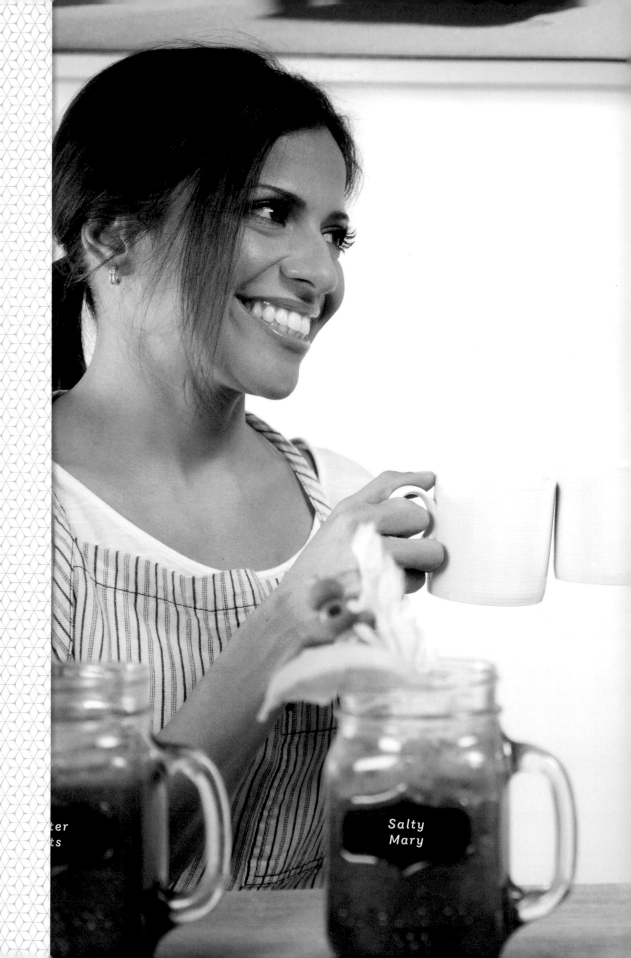

Salty
Mary

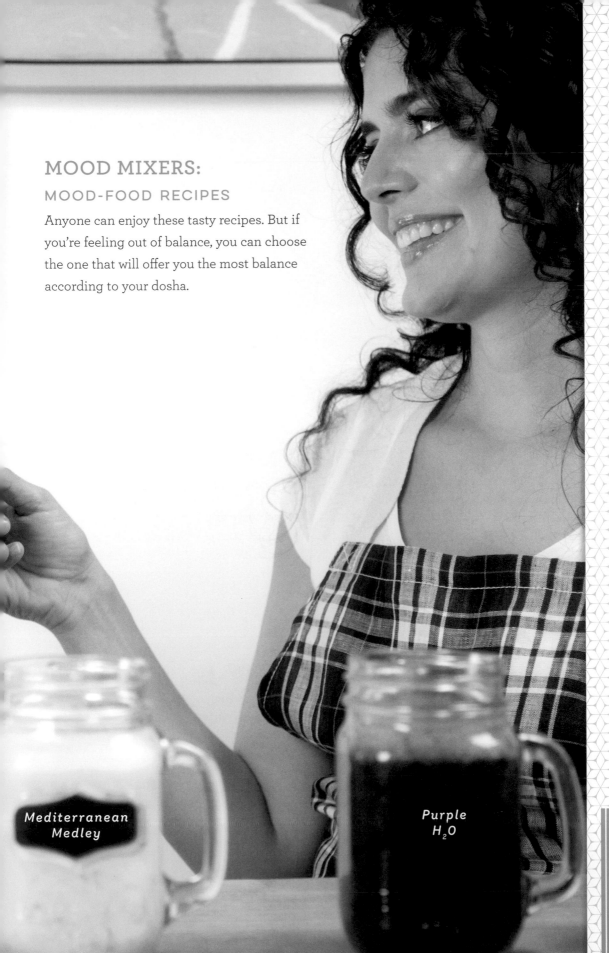

MOOD MIXERS:
MOOD-FOOD RECIPES

Anyone can enjoy these tasty recipes. But if you're feeling out of balance, you can choose the one that will offer you the most balance according to your dosha.

Mediterranean Medley

Purple H$_2$O

Good for balancing Vata and Pitta

INGREDIENTS

1½ cups milk of choice

½ inch fresh ginger cut into small pieces

7 mint leaves

1 tablespoon Darjeeling tea

¼ teaspoon tea masala

2 tablespoons agave syrup

2 dashes ground cardamom

1 dash ground cinnamon

DIRECTIONS

Add all the ingredients into a small pot and bring to a boil. (Milk has a tendency to boil over, so watch your pot.)

Once it comes to a boil, remove the pot from the stove and strain.

Let it cool to the desired temperature or drink hot and enjoy.

SERVING SIZE: 1

⟨ *food for thought*
This special recipe was passed down from my grandparents. My dad swears it cures all moods, and just pouring it makes you feel like royalty. ⟩

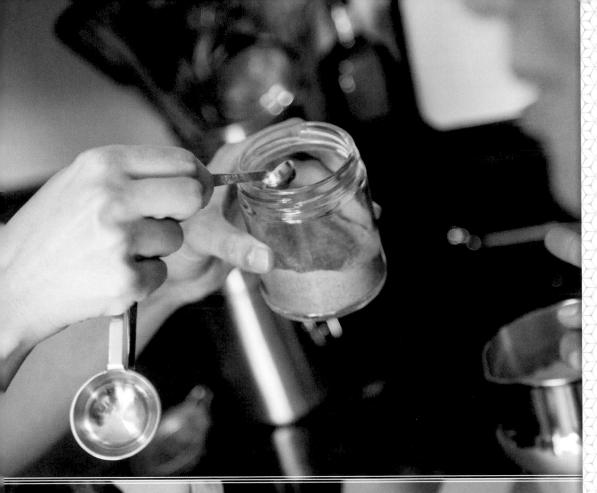

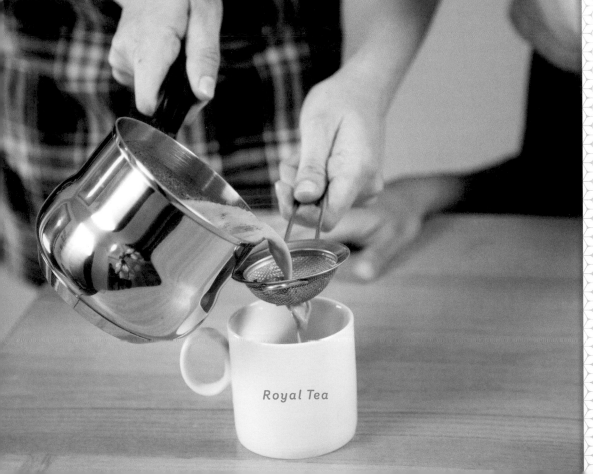

Royal Tea

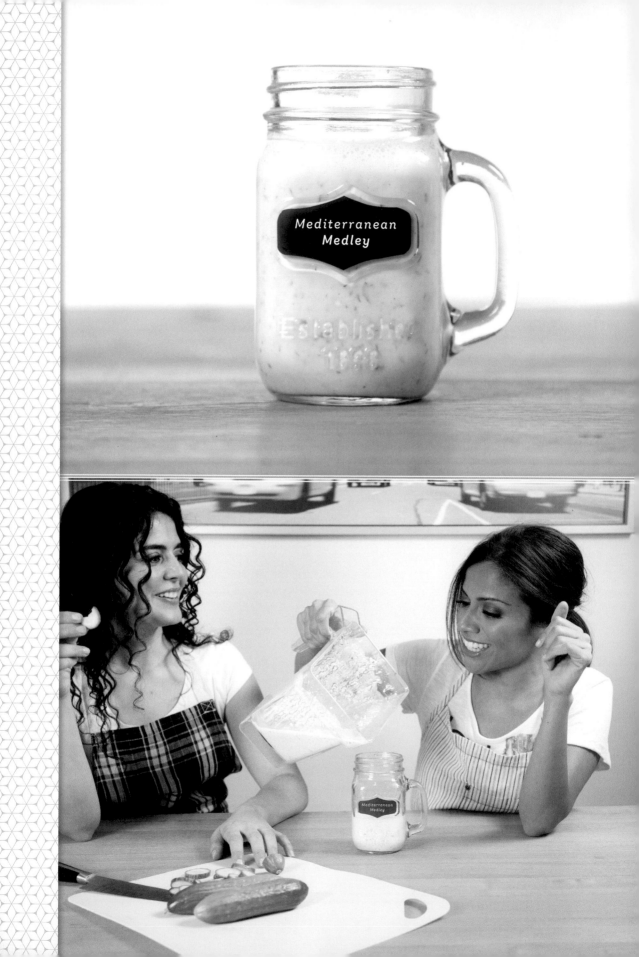

SOUR: *Mediterranean Medley*

Good for balancing Vata

INGREDIENTS

½ cup Persian cucumbers with skin on

1 cup plain Greek yogurt

½ cup water

¼ cup cilantro leaves

¼ teaspoon Himalayan salt

DIRECTIONS

Place all ingredients in a blender and blend until smooth.

Pour and enjoy. (For additional tartness add the juice of ½ lime.)

SERVING SIZE: 1

food for thought

This exotic blend is so refreshing. You'll feel cool as a cucumber whenever you drink it.

SALTY: *Salty Mary*

Good for balancing Vata

INGREDIENTS

¼ cup sliced red bell pepper

½ cup spinach

1 cup tomato juice

½ cup beef broth

1 tablespoon lemon juice

1 teaspoon Worcestershire sauce

3 dashes Tabasco sauce

celery salt to taste

Garnish: Celery, lemon, olives

DIRECTIONS

Place all ingredients in a blender and blend until smooth.

Pour over ice and enjoy.

SERVING SIZE: 1

⟨ *food for thought* ⟩
A Bloody Mary has nothing on this racy mix. Keep the spice and hold the vodka!

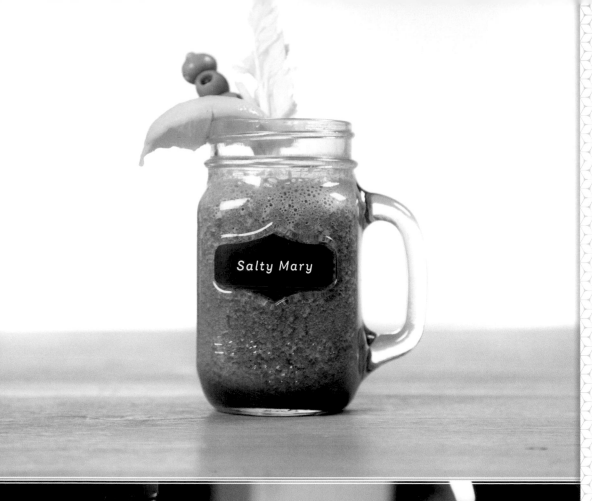

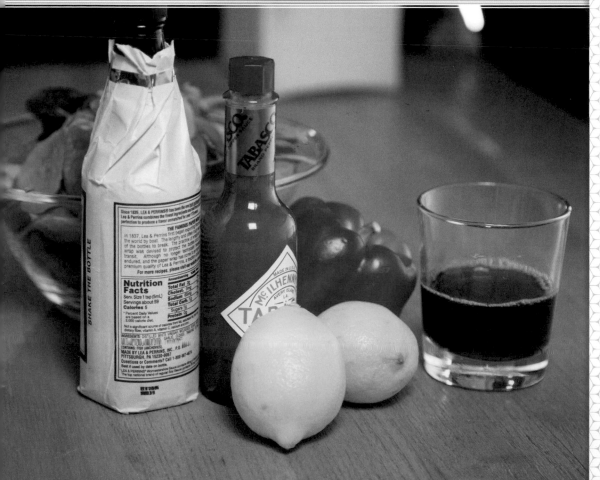

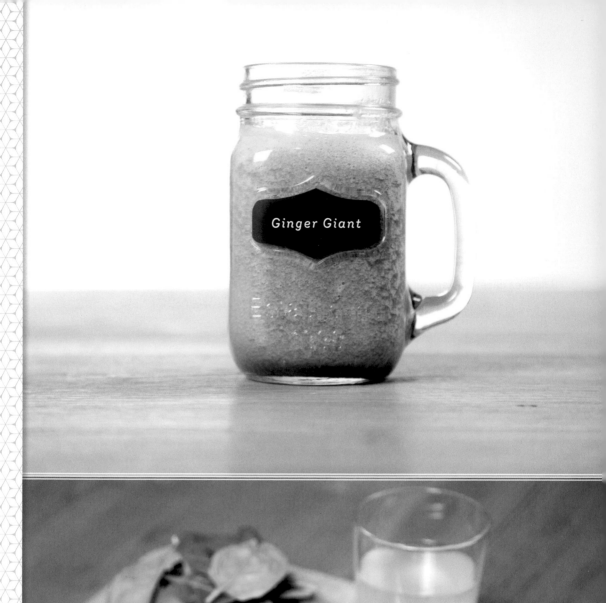

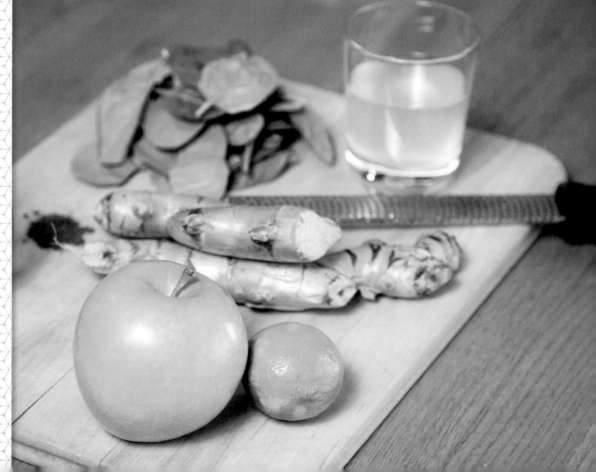

PUNGENT: *Ginger Giant*

Good for balancing Kapha

INGREDIENTS

¾ cup spinach

1 cup sliced apple

1 teaspoon grated ginger

1 cup aloe vera juice with pulp

2 dashes cayenne pepper

½ teaspoon lime juice

DIRECTIONS

Place all ingredients in a blender and blend to desired texture (I like it really smooth).

Strain and enjoy, or for a pulpy texture drink as is.

SERVING SIZE: 1

food for thought

Kick up your step. Ginger packs a punch and all that spinach can stand up to anything.

ASTRINGENT: *Purple H₂O*

Good for balancing Pitta and Kapha

INGREDIENTS

1 cup red seedless grapes

½ cup blueberries

1 cup coconut water (fresh is best!)

DIRECTIONS

Place all ingredients in a blender and blend until smooth or to desired texture.

SERVING SIZE: 1

> *food for thought*
>
> What's better than H_2O? What's better than purple? Answer: Purple H_2O.

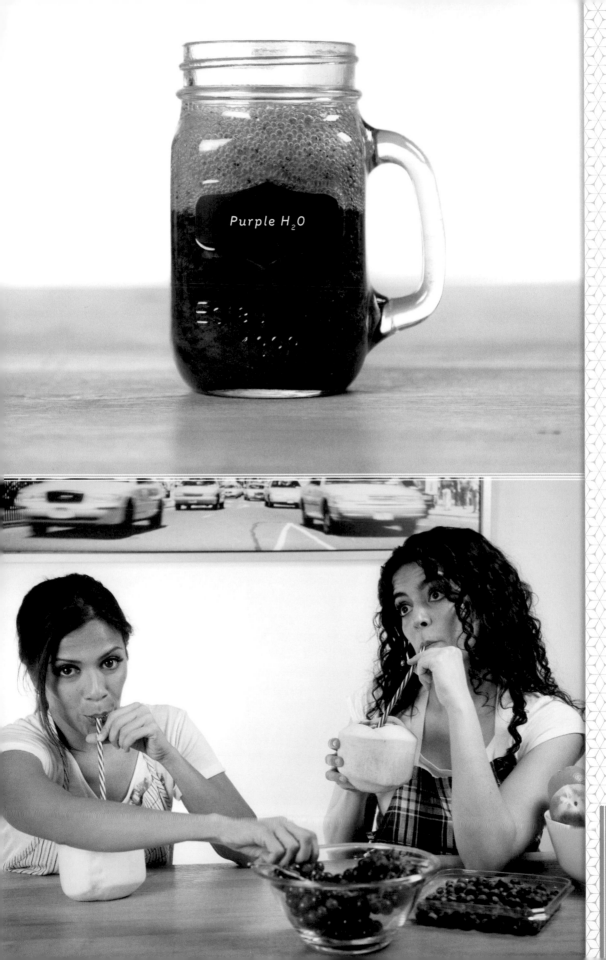

Purple H$_2$O

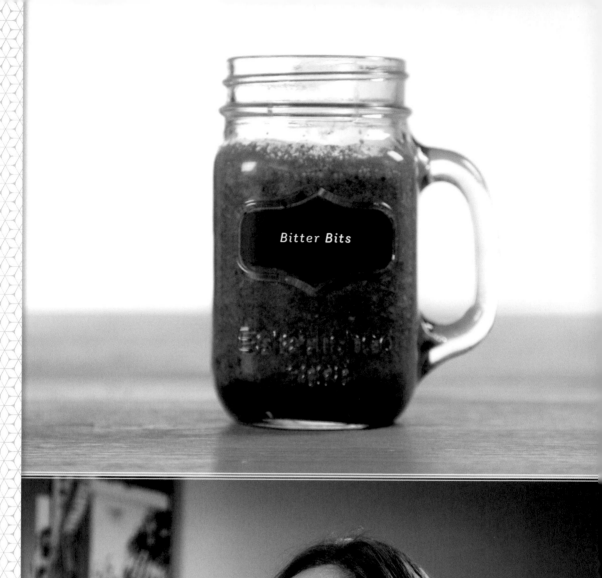

Bitter Bits

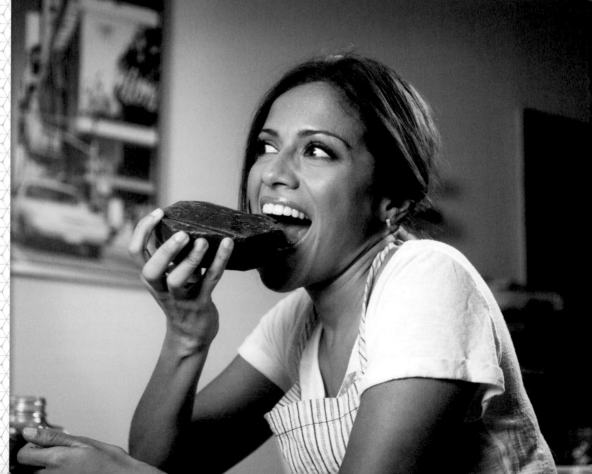

BITTER: *Bitter Bits*

Good for balancing Pitta and Kapha

INGREDIENTS

1 cup pomegranate seeds

¼ cup blackberries

1 cup almond milk

¼ cup shaved 80 percent cacao dark chocolate

DIRECTIONS

Place the pomegranate seeds, blackberries, and almond milk in a blender.

Blend well.

Add the shaved chocolate at the end and pulse blend to desired texture.

Pour and enjoy.

SERVING SIZE: 1

⟨ *food for thought*
Bitter never tasted so good. ⟩

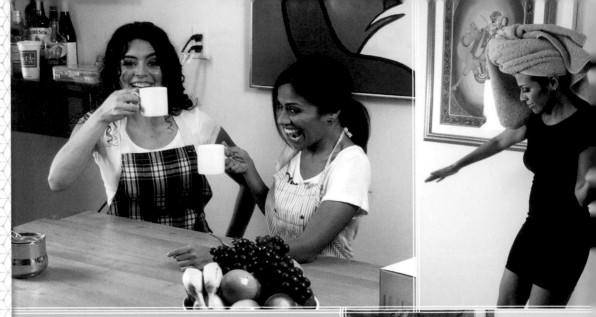

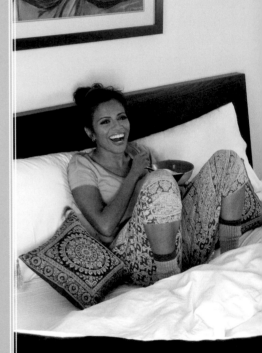

In the Mood for More?

Visit us at nalinimethod.com/bookbonuses
to find resources like these:

Emotional Weight Detox. We've developed
a 6 step detox to help you shed your emotional
weight. Sign up for the complimentary
email course.

Mood Food Recipes. Learn how to prepare
foods that are ideal for your dosha.

Nalini Method Workouts. Sign up to receive
a free month of unique workout routines
full of signature Nalini Method moves!

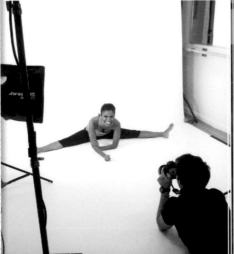

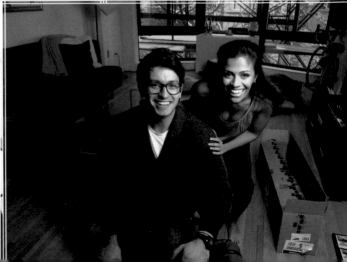

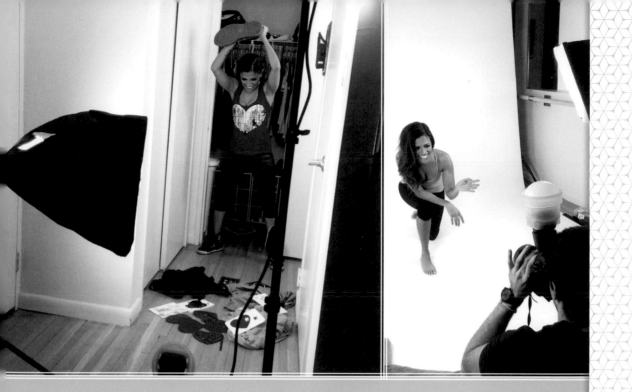

Thank You

Thank you for going on this journey with me and giving me the great opportunity to connect with you. I look forward to hearing about your personal mood journey and workouts.

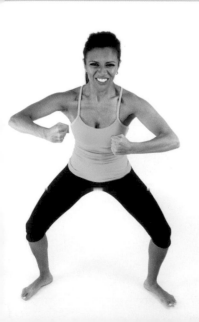

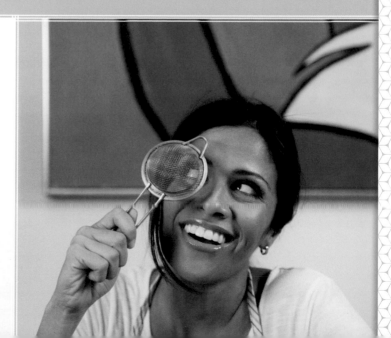

ACKNOWLEDGMENTS

This has been the most difficult page in the book for me to write. I drafted many versions, from a simple quote by Mahatma Gandhi that captures my sentiments to an extensive list of names and experiences that include many blessings, countless acquaintances, friends, family, teachers, schools, businesses, and partners that have greatly impacted the creation and growth of the Nalini Method and NaliniKIDS. I could have written an entire book of just acknowledgments! It's impossible for me to distill a profession so close to my heart and purpose, one that's defined my life, to a handful of names and brief descriptions. But I do want to acknowledge my journey as best I can. And given that two of the greatest gifts I have been given are my *parents* and the *ability to teach*, I'll start there.

My blessed life and dreams would not be possible without my two biggest heroes, my mom and dad. They have been my greatest examples of love and forgiveness, to me and many others, and for that amongst many other lessons, I am forever grateful.

From the people who provided me with the actual studio space to teach, to clients past and present who choose to come to class and share their time with me, to all the school students who open up and work out with me, to current and past coworkers who work relentlessly toward this vision, to old and new partners in the field who have helped promote my business, to reliable friends and family who shower me with encouragement and support, to supporters and collaborators for NaliniKIDS—so many of you have contributed to me having a fulfilling teaching career and businesses pumping with so much heart and purpose.

Many special people from all aspects of my life led me to this book and the mission of the Nalini Method. Listed here are the specific people, part of the current "book crew" that transformed a lifetime of blessings into a tangible book reality. Without the generosity, vision, creativity, intelligence, and work ethic of every one of these individuals, this book would have been impossible.

Alex Glass and **Dan Strone**, agents: I literally wouldn't be writing one word of this if it weren't for both your instincts and your drives. Thank you.

Karen Moline, cowriter: You *are* magic. I am so lucky. Our dynamic feels like high-octane fuel, energizing a passion so close to my heart. Thank you.

Krista Lyons, editor: You believe in me and the message with a smart and patient heart, and for that I am forever grateful. Thank you.

Megan Rynott, copyeditor: Your thoughtful and talented edits made such a huge difference. Thank you.

Laura Mazer, editor: Your warmth and guidance has helped shape not only this book but my confidence. Thank you.

Eva Zimmerman, **Donna Galassi**, and **Anna Gallagher**, publicists: Your bright welcoming of me into your team and your generosity and expertise directly impact my happiness. Thank you.

Jane Musser and **Megan Jones**, designers: Your openness and supportive spirit have made working with you a true pleasure. Thank you.

Roxy Naba, chef and consultant: Meeting you changed my life. You are a true soul sister, and your support and generosity are boundless. Thank you.

Dr. Aparna Bapat, ayurvedic doctor and consultant: You *are* balance, and your patience and wisdom can transform so many. Thank you.

Hannah Kloepfer, content advisor: Because of your strong moral compass, you have quickly become a solid and respected rock in my life. Thank you.

Brandon Fake, content advisor: Your ability to lead and follow, guide and listen, create and support, inspires me every day. Thank you.

Tessa Slovis, content advisor: Your strength, uniqueness, and opinions inspire and dare me to be better. Thank you.

Nidhi Thapar, content advisor: What a great journey we've enjoyed. Your belief in me and patience in teaching me a whole new world are priceless. Thank you.

Liza Summers, content advisor: Our fortunate and timely relationship has provided me with so many gifts in such a short amount of time. I can't wait for what the future holds. Thank you.

Hannah Meadows, teacher: You embody so many admirable traits, and your perseverance and belief in the Nalini Method and me are humbling. Thank you.

Will Haraldson, photographer: If the "Will Haraldson" mood could be a workout, it should be. It's some of the best energy I've been lucky enough to be around. Thank you.

From the beginning to this moment, to everyone, a heartfelt thank-you.

Called a "pint-sized guru" by *Vogue* magazine and the "Rachael Ray of Fitness" by the *New York Post*, **Rupa Mehta** is a teacher, trainer, entrepreneur, philanthropist, and author. As a successful young businesswoman driven to impact children and adults nationwide, she has become an energetic magnet for people wanting to live healthier lives and be more involved with their communities. A first-generation Indian American, Rupa grew up in Fairfax, Virginia, majored in journalism and marketing at New York University, and then received her MBA from the Stern School of Business at New York University. With a passion for helping others find their best emotional and physical selves, Rupa devised her own unique fitness system, the Nalini Method. Noted as "One of the All-time Best Workouts in New York City" by NBC News and voted a Top Workout by *Oprah* and *Fitness* magazines, the Nalini Method is a dynamic workout fusing Pilates, aerobics, barre work, strength and resistance training, and yoga. Rupa's passion is to weave together Eastern and Western philosophies through dynamic and accessible approaches to teaching and wellness. In 2009, partnered with Mayor Bloomberg and NYC Service, Mehta founded her nonprofit organization NaliniKIDS®, a groundbreaking program designed to improve the emotional and physical health of at-risk students in New York City. In partnership with the Department of Education, various charter and private schools, Mehta now trains pre-K–12 school teachers nationwide. NaliniKIDS introduces the first-ever combination of emotional literacy and physical health through the ONE WORD journey. Rupa's one word is *CONNECT*. What's your ONE WORD?

nalinimethod.com
nalinikids.org

— INDEX —

— SELECTED TITLES FROM SEAL PRESS —

Yogalosophy: 28 Days to the Ultimate Mind-Body Makeover, by Mandy Ingber. $20.00, 978-1-58005-445-4. Celebrity yoga instructor Mandy Ingber offers a realistic, flexible, daily plan that will help readers transform their minds, their bodies, and their lives.

The Coregasm Workout: The Revolutionary Method for Better Sex Through Exercise, by Debby Herbenick. $18.00, 978-1-58005-564-2. Fun, fascinating, and useful, *The Coregasm Workout* offers revolutionary new exercise techniques women who want to stay sexy, healthy, and fit, and enjoy the benefits of the gym in the bedroom.

Beautiful You: A Daily Guide to Radical Self-Acceptance, by Rosie Molinary. $16.95, 978-1-58005-331-0. A practical, accessible, day-by-day guide to redefining beauty and building lasting self-esteem from body expert Rosie Molinary.

The 3-Day Reset: Restore Your Cravings For Healthy Foods in Three Easy, Empowering Days, by Pooja Mottl. $22.00, 978-1-58005-527-7. These 10 simple resets target and revamp your eating habits in practical, three-day increments.

What You Can When You Can: Healthy Living on Your Terms, by Roni Noone and Carla Birnberg. $14.00, 978-1-58005-573-4. This companion book to the #wycwyc movement teaches you how to harness the power of small steps to achieve your goals for healthier living.

The Nonrunner's Marathon Guide for Women: Get Off Your Butt and On with Your Training, by Dawn Dais. $17.00, 978-1-58005-205-4. Cheer on your inner runner with this accessible, funny, and practical guide.

Find Seal Press Online
www.sealpress.com
www.facebook.com/sealpress
Twitter: @SealPress